Praise for *On Vanishing*

"[A] searching, poetic inquiry into dementia... [Harper] writes without fear or aversion but with a robust, restless curiosity, a keenness to reframe our understanding of dementia with sensitivity and accuracy... In her beautifully unconventional book, Harper examines the porousness of the borders, the power of imagination and language to grant better futures to our loved ones and ourselves." —PARUL SEHGAL, *The New York Times*

"[A] calm, clear-eyed discussion of new ways to see dementia and its impact on the individual."
—GEMMA TARLACH, *Discover*

"Not many books have so swiftly dismantled my default mode of thinking as Harper's *On Vanishing* . . . Though she writes from sociological and theological perspectives with manifesto-like urgency, *On Vanishing* has the emotional complexity and richness of language of any great work of literary nonfiction. Like the Romantic poets and writers she references throughout, Harper masterfully translates complex abstractions into crystalline distillations . . . An excellent book for anyone, regardless of age or creed, who wants to seriously examine what it means to be mortal." —SOPHIE LEFENS, *Christian Century*

"Lynn Casteel Harper's contemplative new work of nonfiction, *On Vanishing*, [is] a welcome friend . . . Harper asks the reader to reconsider much of the stigma—and terminology—that we place on people diagnosed with dementia . . . [A] meditation, and a lamentation." —JOE PAGETTA, *America: The Jesuit Review of Faith & Culture*

"A moving and deeply compassionate call to action on behalf of the millions of people who live with or care for someone with dementia . . . Harper offers us new ways to understand, appreciate, and interact with people who are by no means 'gone.'" —JESSICA PIERCE, *Zócalo Public Square*

"Harper writes beautifully . . . *On Vanishing* helps us understand what's at stake in healthcare systems that risk prioritizing data collection and cure over medicine as unfolding story . . . Harper shows us how 'vanishing is still life,' filled with sometimes startling surprises worth telling, hearing, and experiencing together." —ROBERT MUNDLE, *Intima*

"Dementia is a catch-all term for different diseases that affect more than 50 million people around the world as they age, leading to memory loss, struggles with language, and a decline in motor skills. Baptist minister Lynn Casteel Harper has seen dementia's impact as she's worked as a chaplain in nursing homes, and in this book, she weaves those experiences with broader research about aging, healthcare, and death to explore how we can bestow more dignity on those who are 'vanishing.'"

—*Bitch*

"A compassionate collection of essays examining dementia from an unusually hopeful point of view . . . Harper moves smoothly between abstract reflections and concrete experiences, reflecting often on the effects of dementia on her grandfather and on her relationship with him, her fears that a genetic link to the disease may have been passed down to her, and her encounters with many individuals, all described in strikingly specific terms, surviving dementia in their own ways . . . Moving insights into a situation many will face."

—*Kirkus Reviews*

"The best nonfiction opens the mind in ways we didn't know it needed to be opened. Lynn Casteel Harper does that and more in *On Vanishing*, a significant contribution to writing on neurodiversity and aging, and a profound and useful corrective to the Western way of thinking about the trajectory of human life. I was afraid of what *On Vanishing* might reveal about my family's future, or mine, or how it might remind me of the suffering of my grandmother. But once I began this important book, I could not put it down or resist quoting it to friends and family. Harper is so wise, compassionate, and hopeful, as are the not-vanished people whose powerful stories she has gathered here."

—BELLE BOGGS, author of *The Art of Waiting*

"*On Vanishing* is imbued with rich humanity, laden with good, orderly directions on the mysteries of age and desolation, and freighted with sentences so beautiful and sad, they catch the breath away. Lynn Casteel Harper's generous text suggests that dementia, apart from the litany of loss it is, might also be, for caregiver and afflicted alike, a chance at love, a way to grow in grace." —THOMAS LYNCH, author of *The Depositions*

"This inspiring work takes us far from our often-arrogant efforts to vanquish (cure) dementia to seeing human vanity in another light. How do we envision vanishing and disappearance in the face of progressive cognitive decline? In *On Vanishing*, Lynn Casteel Harper holds a mirror to society and asks us to reflect . . . Just what does dying with dementia tell us about the human condition, both in the details of individual lives and in the grand scope of society? . . . In these troubled times of environmental deterioration and social injustice, can we learn to create more compassionate civilizations that celebrate caring? —PETER J. WHITEHOUSE, MD, author of *The Myth of Alzheimer's*

"A marvelous tapestry. *On Vanishing* is poignant in its personal history, profound in its understanding, and prophetic in its analysis of the ways social norms, values, and systems shape the lives of people with dementia and their loved ones. What's more, it is beautifully written. My copy is full of underlines and checks, noting quotes I wish I could remember but now

know I can find. Lynn Casteel Harper helps us to see dementia through different sets of eyes, ones that recognize the mystery of our own humanness."
—BILL GAVENTA,
author of *Disability and Spirituality: Recovering Wholeness*

"Elegantly balancing the intimate and the investigative, Lynn Casteel Harper explores the much-feared disease of dementia, opening a compassionate window into territory that is too often simplified and reduced. As an antidote to avoidance and marginalization, this compelling book also takes on broader questions about the relationship between aging and transformation; *On Vanishing* will spark necessarily nuanced conversations within institutions as well as across generations."
—ELIZABETH ROSNER, author of *Survivor Café*

"*On Vanishing* is at once intellectual and soulful, vulnerable and brave. With clear eyes and a steady heart, Harper plumbs the complexities of vanishing—the ways the elderly disappear from society and from this world. Grounded in deep compassion and unwillingness to write off those we so easily forget, Harper's book elaborates a beautifully meditative and often radically progressive inquiry into the experience of mental decline and, ultimately, of being a person who will die." —MARIN SARDY,
author of *The Edge of Every Day: Sketches of Schizophrenia*

On Vanishing

On Vanishing

MORTALITY, DEMENTIA, AND
WHAT IT MEANS TO DISAPPEAR

Lynn Casteel Harper

Catapult
New York

Copyright © 2020 by Lynn Casteel Harper
First paperback edition: 2021

Hardcover ISBN: 978-1-948226-28-8
Paperback ISBN: 978-1-64622-056-4

Cover design by Nicole Caputo
Book design by Wah-Ming Chang

Library of Congress Control Number: 2019946559

Printed in the United States of America
10 9 8 7 6 5 4 3 2 1

To Jack and Edna

Contents

On Vanishing

I

Introduction

WITH VANISHING ON MY MIND, I CROSSED CENTRAL Park to the Metropolitan Museum of Art on a late autumn morning on a sober errand. Ginkgo leaves, freshly fallen, coated my path. My root-word research on "vanishing"—which, like "vanity," comes from the Latin *evanescere* ("die away") and *vanus* ("empty void")—had led me to a genre of still-life painting that flourished in the Netherlands in the early seventeenth century.

The *vanitas* school of painting takes its name from the Latin version of an Ecclesiastes refrain ("Vanity of vanities! All is vanity") and it involves carefully juxtaposing objects deemed symbolic of life's brevity and the evanescence of earthly achievements. Objects such as mirrors, broken or tipped

glassware, books, decaying flowers, and skulls are meant to encourage viewers to contemplate their own mortality. Jacques
de Gheyn's *Vanitas Still Life*, the earliest known *vanitas* painting, hangs in one of the Met's seemingly less popular galleries.
Most visitors pass through this corridor of dark still-life paintings on their way to lighter, more moving pieces. That autumn
morning, I had *Vanitas Still Life* to myself.

A modest-sized piece, 32.5 by 24.25 inches, it contains a pan-
oply of *vanitas* symbols. A thin stream of vapor rises from an urn,
an orange flower with browning leaves languishes in another.
Dutch medals and Spanish coins glitter in the foreground. Two
philosophers—Democritus, the "laughing" philosopher, and
Heraclitus, the "crying" philosopher—recline in the painting's
top corners, pointing to the objects below. A large transparent bubble hovers above a human skull. From every angle, the
viewer confronts images of life's transience, but it is the skull
that serves as the central reminder of human vanishing. The
empty eye sockets locked my gaze, making me think—vainly—
of my own future. A hollowed head, more than any other bodily
remnant, symbolizes death's totality, an unyielding force that
consumes the entire person, even the ability to think. I guess
there's a reason why the sight of Yorick's skull, not his rib cage
or pelvic bone, occasions Hamlet's famous lament.

As a condition associated with the head, dementia—like the *vanitas* skull—ignites an especially acute awareness of mortality,

placing our very selves under death's scrutiny. In the last decade, I have glimpsed dementia from several different angles. I have seen dementia-related deaths in my own family. I have worked with dementia sufferers day-to-day in my capacity as a nursing home chaplain. I recently discovered that both of my parents carry one copy of ApoE4, a gene variant strongly linked to late-onset Alzheimer's disease. I have a 50 percent chance of having a single copy of the gene, which doubles or triples my risk of developing the disease. I have a 25 percent chance of having two copies, which elevates my risk by eight to twelve times, giving me a 51 to 68 percent chance of having Alzheimer's by the time I am eighty-five. My particular bloodlines aside, the chance of getting Alzheimer's disease, the most common form of dementia, is one in nine after age sixty-five and one in three after eighty-five. Nearly six million people in the United States are living with Alzheimer's—making it the nation's sixth leading cause of death. And yet nuanced thinking about dementia is largely absent—perhaps even nonexistent—in public discourse.

Heart disease impairs circulation. Kidney disease impairs filtration. But brain disease impairs communication. By distinctly and directly impacting our abilities to relate with ourselves and others, it confronts us with the *fact* of our humanness: to be human is to be limited, even in our most cherished capacities. Perhaps more than other conditions, dementia brings our fundamental lack of ultimate control over our lives, and their endings, to a head.

Rather than confirming the humanness of sufferers, dementia, curiously, is often viewed as throwing it into question. A gerontologist once told me over lunch that he begins
his dementia caregiver workshops by telling participants that
their loved ones remain persons throughout their illness. He
reminds caregivers that, even as their relatives become more
inaccessible, their "core" never leaves. I am glad for his admo-
nition; I am also troubled that it is needed. I doubt caregivers
of persons with terminal heart disease need such instruction,
or caregivers of infants need reminders that, even though their
babies cannot talk or use the bathroom, they remain people.

That we need reminders that persons living with dementia
are "still people" elevates my curiosity and my suspicion about
the peculiar burdens dementia-causing diseases bear. We seem
to have placed dementia beyond the scope of ordinary human
imagining, as if this condition alone reveals some nasty, shame-
ful secret: the ease with which we all may disappear.

The cultural critic Susan Sontag's classic *Illness as Metaphor*
emerged from her rage at seeing, after her own cancer diagnosis, "how much the very reputation of this illness added to
the suffering of those who have it." In 1978, Sontag contended
with cancer's reputation as scourge, invader, predator, demonic
pregnancy, demonic enemy, barbarian within. Cancer's roots
were then imagined, at least in part, as psychological, result-
ing from repressed emotion. These metaphoric conceptions of

cancer saddled its sufferers with shame and prevented many from seeking proper treatment or even knowing their diagnosis. A decade later, in *AIDS and Its Metaphors*, Sontag turned her critique to popular metaphors surrounding AIDS, the new "scourge," which gravitated toward the language of contagion and contamination, carrying an even greater charge of stigmatization. AIDS, Sontag wrote, was among "grave illnesses regarded as more than just illnesses." It was perceived "not just as lethal but as dehumanizing"; it supposedly degraded and dissolved the person. Sontag hoped that even this disease, so "fraught with meaning," could become, one day, "just an illness."

In our contemporary moment, I think Alzheimer's has become another disease "fraught with meaning." It, too, is regularly spoken of as a force that degrades and dissolves a person. Rather than the fear of invasion or contagion, it evokes the fear of advancing oblivion. The disease is "the long goodbye," people say, or "the death that leaves the body behind." The afflicted become the "living dead," who have vanished in plain sight. We are taught to think that dementia displaces persons, turning their faces to "blank stares" and their bodies to "shells," making strangers of intimates. A thief, kidnapper, slow-motion murderer, Alzheimer's purportedly robs, steals, and erases one's memory, mind, personality—even one's very self. That persons with dementia are so readily envisioned as vanished or vanishing, succumbing to an especially terrifying, slow-moving, unstoppable vortex of suffering, surely speaks to anxieties beyond the ordinary fears of death and disease. The intense negativity of dementia metaphors—combined with their ubiquity—moves them beyond vivid description of brain disease; they express an outsized dread. It seems dementia has become more than just an illness.

I worry that the language we think describes a reality also creates one, that Alzheimer's notorious reputation adds to the suffering of those who have it, their caregivers, and everyone else in the at-risk population—that is, all of us who plan to grow old. Images of vacancy seem to push persons who do not have dementia away from those who do, keeping "us" at arm's length from "them." If "the light's on but nobody's home," why would I (or anyone else) wish to visit?

The story of how I became involved with dementia is not entirely straightforward—perhaps mirroring the oblique course of dementia itself. I can trace some of my interest back to the summer after I began divinity school, the summer I turned twenty-four, when I completed my first unit of chaplaincy training in a hospital. I was reluctant to enroll in the ten-week program, fearing I did not have the constitution for this kind of work. The last time I had been inside a hospital was five years prior, when I had visited a friend who had been in a motorcycle accident. When she described the pins screwed into her hips, I fainted and fell backward, hitting my head on the cold ceramic floor. I spent the afternoon in the emergency room for observation.

But with no other prospects for the summer, I applied to the program, and was assigned to a neurological unit where patients were recovering from brain surgery. They had had tumors, aneurysms, strokes. I spent each day with patients who struggled to find words, to relearn basic tasks, and to just stay awake. I learned about brain death when I was called to the room of a teenage kid who had crashed his four-wheeler into a tree. His mother's knees buckled when she received the news that her son was brain-dead.

The fragility of the brain pressed in upon me, and I began to confront how closely I had tied my sense of identity and worth to my own intellectual ability, a metric that now felt remarkably tenuous. I wanted to push away this disquieting insight, but grappling with the brain's changeability would not leave me so easily. Two weeks after I left the hospital, I began a requisite yearlong internship. My placement was a continuing care retirement community, also known as a CCRC, which, I learned, is a campus that contains tiered levels of care, including independent living, assisted living, and skilled nursing or "nursing home" care. Rather than the acute brain traumas I encountered in the hospital, this assignment exposed me to the ordinary frailties of aging minds.

I shadowed the community's two chaplains—Maurice and Ray. I recall Maurice listening with great attention to a woman with severe dementia. While I could not make any sense of what she was saying, Maurice seemed utterly engaged. Later, he spoke to me about the importance of listening to patients' word fragments and connecting them to Latin morphemes. At the time, I found this lesson a bit tedious and far-fetched, but what strikes me now is how seriously he had taken her, how he had presumed a meaningful interaction was possible. The woman was not lost to all meaning—she needed careful and creative interlocutors and interpreters.

Each week I accompanied Ray to the Memory Enhanced Residence, a small wing of the facility where a dozen or so residents who had dementia lived in a homey environment, with a shared living room and dining table. After Ray read from the Bible and gave a brief reflection, he would ask a resident named Thelma to give the closing prayer. She had been a pastor's wife, and the intonation and fervor of her prayers reflected decades of blessing meals, church meetings, and Sunday school classes. While I did not always follow the logic of her prayers, how one sentiment connected to the next, I sensed their sincerity and the calm assurance that overtook Thelma and that touched me, too.

After I completed my Master of Divinity degree, I began a nine-month chaplain residency program at a New Jersey hospital. One of my three assigned units was in the basement next to the morgue. It was designated for patients who had chronic conditions such as emphysema, who were not acute enough for the ICU but not stable enough to go home. Most of these patients were old. As the year progressed, the unit began to house mentally ill patients who had come to the emergency room and were waiting to be transferred to a psychiatric hospital. Physically frail old people and psychologically fragile adults of all ages were lumped together in the bleak, remote bowels of the hospital—a sad picture of the wider culture's exclusion of these same populations. Perhaps this combination of patients was preparing me to understand some of the stigma around older persons with dementia. I spent a disproportionate amount of my time on this unit, finding many of its occupants starved for human encounter beyond what was clinically expedient or cognitively normative. Regular back-and-forth conversation held little comfort for many of these patients, who did not have the energy or attention for words.

A few months after I completed the residency, I was hired as the chaplain at a 1,400-resident CCRC on the New Jersey Shore. The campus contained eight buildings of independent living apartments, connected by hallways and a sky bridge, and one five-story building of assisted living and skilled nursing rooms. I served the residents who lived in this latter facility, called the Gardens, which sat on the edge of campus, detached from the rest of community. It was here where my specific passion for persons with dementia and for the philosophical and spiritual issues surrounding the mind's vulnerability was forged.

On my first day at the Gardens—the first day of nearly seven years—an administrator gave me a tour of each of the five floors. The only part of the tour I recall is my introduction to the fourth floor, a skilled nursing unit that had been designated for residents with severe dementia. I have a hazy memory of stepping just inside the doorway of the unit's large activity room. A young staff member, wearing a Hawaiian shirt and floppy straw hat, supported an old man by the elbow as he lumbered across the room. I do not recall with clarity any other individuals who filled the room that day, only wheelchairs and slumped bodies. My guide told me that I would likely not spend much time here. With nearly two hundred residents under my care, I would find other (better, more productive) ways to fill my day than visiting persons who would forget me the moment I left.

Memory is tricky. I now wonder if he had indeed expressed his prejudices to me directly, or if I absorbed them indirectly, or if I simply carried them within myself. Nevertheless, I received a clear message, consistent with a dementia-phobic culture: my presence would not be needed with these particular residents, my absence would not be noticed. The unspoken corollary: *I* would not need these persons' presence or be impacted by *their* absence. They were considered to have disappeared from themselves, and I was expected to disappear from them.

In 2014, I left the Gardens and moved to South Carolina, where my husband had accepted a two-year visiting academic appointment. During this period, I feverishly read and wrote about dementia and spirituality. I also began facilitating occasional workshops on the subject, as faith groups asked me for help in relating to their congregants with dementia. Populated mostly by professional and family caregivers, these workshops have kept me in direct dialogue with people who are intimately invested in the lives of persons who have dementia. After my husband's position ended in 2016, we moved to New York City, where I became the minister of older adults at the Riverside Church, a large interracial, interdenominational congregation in Upper Manhattan. Working with elders at the church, as well as leading workshops, continues to connect me to issues surrounding brain aging. But it was my time at the Gardens, which overlapped with the last years of my grandfather's life with dementia, that served as the crucible in which this book was formed.

The closer I came to people with dementia, the more my assumptions vanished, the more they became individuals rather than a blur of disability. While I encountered diminishment and loss on the Gardens' dementia unit, there was more than just deterioration. At times I felt I was witnessing, instead, a kind of ascendency—of compassion, honesty, humility. I befriended Evelyn, a retired math teacher, who spoke to me as a colleague, often asking, "How are your students?" I met Mary, who, despite her acute anxiety, readily assisted her less-mobile neighbors, pushing them in their wheelchairs to activities and meals—and who once helped me plan a party. I met Bernice, who taught me that not all of the disappearances associated with dementia prove unwelcome or tragic. What vanished in Bernice's later years were some of the distressing manifestations of her long-standing mental illness. Crippling anxiety and paranoid delusions gave way to more laughter and delight. One day she pointed out my gray hair, grinned, and declared, "See, you're aging, too! Just like us!"

I came to know these residents and so many more—not primarily as defective victims of Alzheimer's, presumed to be "lost" to their disease—but as complex, dynamic individuals. And I began to wonder: why do *we*—those whom the dementia activist Morris Friedell termed the "temporarily able-brained"—need *them* to vanish? Why are we so eager to view them as disappearing or disappeared? And what possibilities are we precluding, what hard work of the soul are we avoiding, by imposing this distance?

I want to probe the distance. I want to understand why certain metaphors dominate, eclipsing other ways of imagining dementia, and how these depictions of dementia generate and reinforce stigma. I want to interrogate the cultural, social, political, and spiritual values that disproportionately define us by certain cognitive capacities. I am searching for new, more robust renderings of dementia that expand our vision beyond progressive vacancy and dread.

It was Betty who originally stretched my imagination. In my first months at the Gardens, Betty helped initiate me to the fourth floor's rich potential. She always carried a floppy, well-worn Bible on her lap, as she wheeled herself up and down the unit's hallways. When I suggested to Betty that she and I start a Bible study on the floor, she happily agreed. On Thursday afternoons, with a few of her neighbors, we began to gather in a small dining room across from the common room. I had no idea what to do, so I began at the beginning, reading stories from Genesis. Betty, who kept her eyes closed most of the time, came forth with great insights and funny quips, but only after she had sat in silence for many minutes. On the afternoon I read the story of Joseph's brothers throwing him in a pit and selling him into slavery, she exclaimed, "Oh, the jealousy!" as the other participants were dispersing after our closing prayer. I learned that her long silences did not mean she was disengaged. She taught me to slow down and wait with my mouth shut.

Like any good evangelical, Betty lamented that the group was not bigger; she wanted converts, new recruits. She had imagined throngs, not just three or four acquaintances in a small circle. Her passion for engaging others struck me as utterly loving, a thoroughly intact desire to reach beyond herself. Betty's tireless energy laid the groundwork for the group to flourish after her death. Although perhaps not quite in the way she would have hoped, the group did grow, evolving into an interfaith spirituality group of nine or ten devoted attendees. Our meetings became the highlight of my week. Whether facilitating this group, visiting with residents and their families, or chatting with stretched-thin staff, I found I spent more time on this floor than any other.

The Buddhist nun Pema Chödrön says we work on ourselves in order to help others, and we help others in order to work on ourselves. We go into the areas of society that we have rejected so we can reconnect with the parts of ourselves we have rejected. I spent time on the dementia unit not because I was some kind of martyr or saint, or because the work came preternaturally easily to me (it did not), but because, perhaps, I sensed I could mature as a minister—as a person—only if I learned how to embrace those people whom we can all too easily believe have nothing to offer. Perhaps, in the process of knowing them, I might come to embrace the seemingly unworthy—confused, strange, fragmented—parts of myself. If my faith was supposed to culminate in cheerful bedside conversations, erudite sermons, eloquent prayers, unending activities and activism, and word-heavy worship services, then I (and the larger tradition of which I am a part, as a Baptist minister in the mainline Protestant vein) would have little or nothing to learn from persons with dementia, and even less to offer them. But I began to see my faith—and my role—in different terms. I think dementia—the process of turning it over in my mind, investigating it, and above all, coming close to persons living with it—has slowly stretched my imagination about spirituality, asking me to value silence and absence, to embrace strangeness and spontaneity, to revere the nonverbal and nonlinear.

Around the time I began working at the Gardens, my own family was encountering up-close the depths of dementia. On the morning of my grandparents' weekly shopping trip, the teenage boy whom my mother had hired to shuttle her parents around town found my grandfather on the lawn mower and my grandmother unresponsive in bed. Apparently, unable to rouse his wife of sixty-five years, my grandfather had gone outside to mow the lawn.

My grandmother's sudden death exposed the hundreds of ways she had compensated and covered for my grandfather's dementia. What we had dismissed as hearing loss, a bout of depression, or a touch of senility, revealed itself as something progressive and pervasive. Overnight, my mother became his caregiver. My mother and her father were living in an intimate way what I was encountering in a professional setting half a country away. Unlike me, they did not leave the dementia floor at five every evening; they were grounded in the round-the-clock realities.

During the year I began writing this book, and just a few months after I had left the Gardens, my grandfather died. This book, in part, seeks to trace the long shadow of his absence and to honor and reframe his presence. But, ultimately, it is not *about* him. While I hope this book sheds light on how to better care for people with dementia, my primary aim does not involve teaching techniques or methods. Rather, this book is about those of us who do not have dementia yet; those of us who never will; and those of us who are already suffering dementia's effects or have friends or family who are. It is about examining our fears, questioning our culture, and—at least in my case—reorienting one's spirituality in light of the challenges and possibilities such diseases bring forth. It is a book about vanishing, and what "vanishing" really means.

The skull in *Vanitas Still Life*, while undoubtedly grim, bears a wry, gapped grin—a grin missing four front teeth. Stripped of its flesh, our bone structure apparently discloses a faint, effortless smile. The skull's stark, denuded presence signals gravity, but its blithe affect signals buoyancy. Perhaps this face of death reflects both the weeping Heraclitus and the laughing Democritus, pointing viewers back to Ecclesiastes: there is "a time to weep and a time to laugh." Wisdom here comes lodged in apposition—pairs of apparent opposites, united by the word "and": "a time to be born, and a time to die [. . .] a time to break down, and a time to build up [. . .] a time to cast away stones, and a time to gather stones together [. . .]" These lines in Ecclesiastes encourage readers to imagine a world in which the poles of existence create vibrant tension, in which life and death, gathering and releasing, embracing and refraining, weeping and laughing, do not negate each other, but instead balance and enrich. There is aggregation and integration—even with loss, even in death.

Dementia, too, invites this kind of conjunction. There is dilution and distillation, constriction and expansion, disorder and constancy. Certain aspects of persons and their relationships fade—and other dimensions crystallize, possessing a new kind of clarity. Dementia places new constraints on communication—and relationships expand to include new ways of being and loving. Cognitive changes upset the usual patterns of one's life—and some rhythms remain unchanged.

I heard a woman describe her spouse with dementia as "my gone but not gone husband," and her phrase seemed to strike at the heart of dementia's paradoxes: an acute awareness of absence, and an equal insistence on presence. Lately, I am struck by its general relevance, as I consider my own gone and not-gone self. The cells that comprise my body—all of our bodies—routinely break down or slough off, and new ones take their place. Some cells, like neurons, die and are never replaced. Paradox lives at the heart of my faith, too: the gone and not-gone ego, the gone and not-gone Jesus. The play of presence and absence infuses all of life, I think, both before and after dementia.

Maybe if we can learn to inhabit this tension, this space between opposites, then dementia and the lives it touches can rejoin the spectrum of human experience, rather than being reduced to tired tropes and burdened by outsized fears, its sufferers and caregivers made to disappear. Imagine if we received *all* lives—those with and without dementia—as conglomerations of the ordinary and the peculiar, the fragmented and the whole, the present and the vanishing.

2

On Vanishing

I HAVE OFFICIATED ONLY ONE MEMORIAL SERVICE IN which I thought the dead person might come back. Dorothy was 103, and she was known for surprise reappearances. Dorothy had resided in an independent living apartment at the retirement community, and I had visited her on the few occasions when she had come to the Gardens to recover from an illness. I had learned over the course of these visits that as a teenager, she had left home to become a stage assistant to Harry Houdini—against her parents' wishes, of course. What did a nice Methodist girl, a preacher's daughter, want with an older man—a Vaudeville magician, no less—rumored to be a Jew, the son of a rabbi? Only after Houdini and his wife, Bess, visited Dorothy's parents and promised to care for her as their own daughter did her parents relent.

In Houdini's shows, Dorothy would pop out from the top of an oversized radio that Houdini had just shown the audience to be empty, kicking up one leg and then the other in Rockette-style extension. Grabbing her at the waist, Houdini would lower her to the floor, where she would dance the Charleston. In another act, she was tied, bound feet to neck, to a pole. A curtain would fall to the floor, and *voila!*—she would reappear as a ballerina with butterfly wings, fluttering across the stage. At the end of each night's performance, Dorothy stood just off stage next to Bess to witness Houdini's finale: the Chinese Water Torture Cell. A shackled Houdini was lowered, upside down, into a tank of water from which he escaped two minutes later. Dorothy knew how he accomplished this stunt—what was often deemed his "greatest escape"—but she never broke confidence.

Dorothy was the last surviving member of Houdini's show. Long after his death, she attended séances on Halloween, awaiting communication with the Great Houdini—which, apparently, was never forthcoming. Eighty-five years after Houdini's death, now she, too, had died. Each time I had visited her, I had felt her end was imminent. Already a petite woman, she seemed to grow smaller and smaller, until I was sure I would find her one day simply gone. But somehow she persisted—until she died about three years into my tenure.

As I prepared for her memorial, I imagined her doing one

of her famous acts at the service. Instead of an oversized radio, her legs would kick open and emerge—up one, up two—from a once-closed coffin. Back to do the Charleston one last time. Or, breaking free from the chains of death, she would pirouette through the parlor in her butterfly wings. Instead, her son, who was in his eighties and also lived at the retirement community, opted for a casketless memorial service rather than a traditional funeral, and this somewhat allayed my anxieties about the coffin popping open. While a reappearance out of thin air seemed less likely, I knew by then that anything was possible with her.

Dorothy went to her grave without ever having revealed Houdini's secrets, true to the vow she took at seventeen. I wonder what it is like to hold the keys to illusion, to know how to unbind one's self, to learn the mechanisms of vanishing, to feel the weight of magic's wisdom. Had she not been so scrupulously loyal, perhaps she could have helped the rest of us solve the riddle of how to vanish well.

•

I came of age in the 1990s when terms like "the right to die," "persistent vegetative state," and "advance directive" infused public discourse, and debates raged over euthanasia. In grade school, I became vaguely aware of Nancy Cruzan, a resident of my home state of Missouri, and Terri Schiavo—women who could not articulate their end-of-life wishes, whose bodies became the site of fierce political contestation. Dr. Jack Kevorkian was solidly a household name. In defiance of the law, he had helped dozens of seriously ill patients end their lives. His visage saturated the media, even appearing on a 1993 cover of *Time* with the title "Doctor Death" and the question "Is he an angel of mercy or a murderer?" It was only recently, however, that I learned of Kevorkian's first client, a fifty-four-year-old English teacher from Portland, Oregon, named Janet Adkins. Diagnosed with early-onset Alzheimer's disease, she could and did articulate her wishes and decided to make herself gone before the disease got the chance.

At a press conference shortly after his wife's death, Ron Adkins read from Janet's suicide note: "I have decided for the following reasons to take my own life. This is a decision taken in a normal state of mind and is fully considered. I have Alzheimer's disease and do not want to let it progress any further. I do not want to put my family or myself through the agony of this terrible disease." One week after beating her sons at tennis, according to reports, she lay supine in the back of Kevorkian's 1968 VW van in a parking lot in a Detroit suburb. In her arm: an IV hooked to the pathologist's own invention, the Thanatron, which delivered heart-stopping potassium chloride into her bloodstream.

Janet Adkins's sympathizers pointed to the horrific prospect of this dementing disease's pathology and her calculated courage. While she could still act on her own behalf, in what she had called in her note a "normal state of mind," Janet Adkins headed off what she imagined as agony for her future self and her family. A pianist, Janet Adkins feared losing music, reportedly telling her pastor, "I can't remember my music. I can't remember the scores. And I begin to see the beginning of the deterioration and I don't want to go through with that deterioration." Perhaps the scores might degenerate into strung-out smudges of black, and she might find notes tangled, unable to fight themselves free to make melody. Perhaps her deterioration would be depleting in every way; it would be saturated with sorrow; it would require heroic fortitude. Perhaps her family would be drained in Sisyphean service to a Janet Adkins unable even to thank them. I imagine Janet Adkins wished to spare her loved ones the torment of her slow self-disappearance.

In the days leading up to Dorothy's service, I read the tributes to her that appeared in major newspapers. I learned that she was the last of two hundred women to audition for Houdini's show and had instantly dazzled the illusionist. After her contract with Houdini had ended, she went on to create a Latin dance called the "rumbalero" and to appear in several movies, including *Flying Down to Rio* with Fred Astaire. In her later years, she donated $12.5 million to build an arts center.

Reading these tributes prompted me to consider the story of my grandfather Jack, whose life—while not as glamorous as Houdini's assistant's—had seemed remarkable to me in its own right. A World War II veteran, Jack received the Distinguished Flying Cross for rescuing a fellow pilot by making a tricky, unauthorized landing in the Himalayas. Upon his return from the war, Jack had considered becoming a band teacher but instead pursued a career in medicine. He played jazz trombone in dive bars at night to pay for medical school. Jack was a committed and smart country doctor. He made house calls and forgave patients' debts. He delivered babies and aided the dying. In the days before defibrillators, Jack once frayed a lamp cord, plugged it in, and shocked a patient to revive him. In retirement, he owned and helped to operate a local pharmacy. Jack was an avid hobbyist—always working in his woodshed or on his computer or on perfecting his omelets. He traveled the world as an ambassador with Rotary International. He maintained his passion for music, singing solos at church, playing the electric organ for his grandkids, and leading songs at Rotary meetings well into his eighties.

The Jack of all these activities—and the Jack who had the ability to narrate them and their importance to him—steadily vanished in his final years. On his eightieth birthday, eleven and a half years before his death, he could not keep score in a simple dice game we played. This singular memory helps me to date the duration of his dementia. At the time of Dorothy's death, Jack was living in an assisted living facility that specialized in memory care. Jack would soon thereafter move to a nursing home where he lived his last two years. If not in bed, he was in his wheelchair at a table with other old war veterans in wheelchairs. He said very few words.

When I told a minister friend about my grandfather's move

to the nursing home, she reflexively responded: *Oh, so he's gone.* Her words reminded me of another friend, who told me that she promised her father that if he ever gets dementia, not to worry, she will take him on a "nice walk to the edge of a cliff." She then made a quick pushing motion—*gone*. It seems persons with dementia are more subject to being pronounced gone— to being pushed off the proverbial cliff—than persons with other kinds of progressive illnesses. While my grandfather's life, in many respects, had "shrunk," he certainly was not gone to those who knew and loved him. But I felt the push toward his erasure, and I wanted to know who or what was doing the pushing.

A couple of weeks after Dorothy's memorial service, I attended a workshop on spirituality and dementia, where I first learned of the late British social psychologist Tom Kitwood, who, in the 1980s and '90s, had developed a new model for providing care to persons with dementia. Challenging the old culture of care that viewed dementia patients as problems to be managed, as bodies in need of physical care and little else, Kitwood argued that people with dementia should be engaged with as complex individuals living within complex social environments. From what I gleaned at the workshop, I sensed that his approach to dementia might help me better understand what contributes to the invisibility of persons with dementia.

In the coming months, I read his seminal work, whose title

alone attracted me: *Dementia Reconsidered: The Person Comes First.* It seemed telling that a reconsideration of dementia would entail something as seemingly obvious as centering the person— as giving persons preeminence in their own lives. Most of the research on dementia had ignored the impact of the social environment on people with dementia, and on their disease process. Kitwood offered a profound corrective. He observed the ubiquity of what he called "malignant social psychology" in relation to persons with dementia. Through close observation of daily interactions between caregivers and dementia patients, Kitwood identified seventeen malignant elements that promote the depersonalization of persons with dementia: treachery, disempowerment, infantilization, intimidation, labeling, stigmatization, outpacing, invalidation, banishment, objectification, ignoring, imposition, withholding, accusation, disruption, mockery, disparagement.

Kitwood argued that care settings shaped by malignant social psychology can actually accelerate neurological decline. He critiqued the "standard paradigm" of dementia, which in his view often blamed only the organic progression of dementia for the decline that sufferers experience. The silent, stigmatizing partner in this dynamic—that is, the cultural bigotry against both cognitive impairment and old age—gets off scot-free. The process of dementia, according to Kitwood, involves "a continuing interplay between those factors that pertain to neuropathology *per se*, and those which are social-psychological." Herein lies the frightening and hopeful prospect: the person with dementia does not simply disappear on her own. It is not just a matter of the private malfunctioning of her private brain. It has to do with *our* malfunctioning, our diseased public mind.

Not long after I read Kitwood, I walked into the program room and found Ruth yelling and pounding her fists on the table. She had recently moved to the dementia unit, where I had met her a few days before during my rounds. At that time, Ruth had been unhappy about her move but not distraught like she was now. Seeing my shock, an activities staff member explained, "She's been terrible to us—yelling out bad things at everyone who walks by. She said she was hungry, that she wanted lunch. But she just ate lunch, so I got her pudding for a snack. And she threw the pudding at me, and it splattered all over the floor. Then she called me a bad name. I'm done; I'm just done." She turned her back to Ruth and walked away.

Understanding Kitwood's malignant social psychology helped me unpack this brief encounter. There was *infantilization*: Ruth was not permitted the food of her choice, because she "just ate lunch." There was *ignoring* and *objectification*: the staff member talked over and about the resident as if she were not there, as if she were a nonentity. There was *imposition*: overriding Ruth's stated desire, the worker insisted she must have a snack instead of a meal. There was *disparagement*: the staff member was clearly angry with Ruth, blaming her for her bad mood. There was *withholding* and *banishment*: the staff member left Ruth, declaring, "I'm just done." Ruth was left alone. Malignancy now hemmed her in. I watched a dining room staff member approach Ruth. "What would you like?" he asked. "A sandwich or something," she replied. He returned from the kitchen with a peanut butter and jelly sandwich. Ruth immediately bit into it. "Thank you, I never thought I'd be this happy with a peanut butter and jelly sandwich," she said.

By this relatively simple act, the staff member had unraveled a bit of the malignancy, but the task of undoing malignant social psychology cannot rest only on direct caregivers. Kitwood understood malignant social psychology as "in the air"—part of our cultural inheritance, not a phenomenon to be blamed on (or solely remediated by) individual caregivers. Malignant responses to dementia, in Kitwood's analysis, revealed tragic inadequacies in our culture, economy, and medical system, which often define a person's worth in terms of financial, physical, and intellectual power.

That certain mental powers determine one's moral standing reflects what the bioethicist Stephen Post calls our culture's "hypercognitive" values, a phrase he first used in his 1995 book, *The Moral Challenge of Alzheimer Disease*. Revisiting the concept in a 2011 article, Post highlights the "troubling tendency," in our hypercognitive culture, to "exclude human beings from moral concern while they are still among the living." Our particular veneration of cognitive acumen generates "dementism"—a term Post uses to describe the prejudice against the deeply forgetful.

Transcending the acts and intentions of discrete individuals, systemic dementism exists in structures that overlook, minimize, or actively undermine the needs of persons with dementia. For example, assisted living facilities, in which approximately seven out of ten residents have some degree of cognitive impairment, are underregulated—leaving people with dementia particularly vulnerable. A severe shortage in the United States of geriatricians, who are often best equipped to provide ongoing clinical support for older persons with dementia, signals a prejudice in the medical system.

The overuse of psychotropic drugs, which carry risky side effects for elders with dementia, is another sign of dementism. Unlike medicines used to treat the cognitive symptoms of dementia, these psychotropic drugs, which include antidepressants, antipsychotics, anxiolytics for anxiety, and antiseizure medications, are used to manage certain behaviors associated with dementia—and are not approved by the FDA for this specific use. Antipsychotic medications are particularly hazardous for older adults with dementia, greatly increasing the likelihood of stroke and death. A study published in 2016 in *International Psychogeriatrics* revealed that only 10 percent of psychotropic drug use among people with dementia is fully appropriate. And yet pharmaceutical companies have pushed the use of such medications for persons with dementia. In 2013, Johnson & Johnson paid a $2.2 billion settlement for the improper promotion of Risperdal, a drug designed to treat schizophrenia and bipolar disorder, for use with dementia patients, despite the company's knowledge of its serious health risks for this population.

As I consider religious institutions within my own Protestant circles, I notice how rarely seminaries offer much if any training to future pastors about aging and dementia. Churches often pump tremendous resources into ministries for young families and children, with little attention to elders—let alone elders with dementia. Progressive churches like mine, which faithfully fight for racial, gender, and economic justice, often fail to take into account ageism and the plight of people with cognitive impairment. Redressing malignant social psychology is not as easy as serving peanut butter and jelly sandwiches. Remediation is needed at every level.

It occurs to me that the possible roots of dementism may lie in a discomfort related to the body; I sense that our culture is fearful both of the body's powerlessness and its power. As I prepared for Dorothy's memorial service, I reflected on such corporeal conundrums. The body is unwieldy and dies. A source of perpetual conflict, the body is at once our home— there's no escaping it—and our battleground, as we struggle to break free from its inevitable demise. We want the box to pop open to reveal our still-kicking legs; we want to shed impossible shackles.

I suspect those bodies in need of hands-on care by others are objects of cultural contempt, because they lay bare our collective fear of the body's fragility and dependence. Perhaps those bodies most charged with the hands-on care of these bodies also bear the taint. The same malignant forces that marginalize the old and the cognitively impaired also marginalize their caregivers, who are often the most economically vulnerable and politically invisible people in American society.

The philosopher Eva Kittay notes that the particular demands of caregiving and the traditional relegation of this work to women or servants make care workers "more subject to exploitation than most." According to a 2018 report released by the Paraprofessional Health Institute, nursing assistants who work in nursing homes—the majority of whom are women of color—suffer workplace injuries at nearly three and a half times the national average. Half of nursing assistants have no formal education beyond high school, and nearly 40 percent rely on some form of public assistance. Fifteen percent of nursing assistants live below the federal poverty line, compared to 7 percent of all U.S. workers.

Nursing assistants spend more time with residents than any other clinical staff, providing a median of 2.2 hours of hands-on care per resident per day. That this occupation, so central to resident care, is both hazardous and poorly compensated reflects the low cultural value placed upon those who perform it and, by extension, their clients. I can count on one hand the occasions I saw administrators on the Gardens' dementia unit spending time with residents and staff. This absence reflected and reinforced the broader culture of invisibility. Perhaps it is little surprise that both the vulnerable staff (often black immigrant women) and their patients (often immobile, voiceless, dependent) were relegated to the same space. The curtain is drawn, hiding them from view—a vanishing act with no scheduled reappearance.

•

Accompanying Dorothy's obituary, many newspapers included a black-and-white photograph of her popping out of Houdini's oversized radio—a prop that looked to me like nothing more than a coffin with dials affixed to it. Next to this box stood a tuxedo-clad, wild-eyed Houdini, his arms agape, holding a wand overhead as he presented his assistant, the "Radio Girl."

The image made me think—perhaps irreverently—of the stories of Jesus's empty tomb and the play of presence and absence that permeated early accounts surrounding his death. In Mark's gospel, when women come to the tomb to anoint Jesus's dead body, a young man dressed in a white robe—presumably an angel—appears to them and points to absence: to nothing but a heap of empty grave clothes. "Look, there is the place they laid him," he says. The women look at where the body *was*. Offered only a brief explanation of the absence—"He has been raised; he is not here"—the women are granted no positive confirmation of Jesus's whereabouts. They respond the way any God-fearing people would: they flee the scene, deathly afraid.

The scene has the right components of a magic show—an expectation of presence or absence (depending upon the setup) and a surprise reversal. I imagined Houdini at Jesus's tomb wearing a white tuxedo and waving a magician's wand overhead as he presented the empty space. The reversal, however, is askew, or it is, at least, incomplete. The dead body should be revealed as *alive*—not merely as missing. But the original ending of Mark, the earliest Gospel, includes no post-resurrection sightings of Jesus. The women at the tomb were to believe based on what was *not* there—a faith based on disappearance.

Uncomfortable with this silence and with the last image being one of women fleeing in fear—and perhaps intuiting the failed dramatic arc—Mark's earliest editors added post-resurrection encounters with Jesus in the flesh, and not just with the clothes his flesh had once inhabited. The later Gospels chronicled rather detailed meetings between the risen Jesus and the disciples. Jesus shows them his feet, hands, and side; he walks through closed doors, breathes on them, and makes breakfast for them on the seashore. In John's Gospel, Mary Magdalene mistakes the risen Jesus for a gardener, until he speaks her name. The disciples experience, with their senses, a newly constituted but still bodily Jesus—and thus gain what we moderns might call a sense of "closure" in the wake of Jesus's traumatic death. When all seems lost, a magical, fleshly reappearance defies death's despair.

Nevertheless, I am drawn to Mark's original ending; it rings truer in light of the abundant absence that, to my mind, marks all earthly existence. The dead don't often visit us again (imagine the silence at the yearly Houdini séance). The Population

Reference Bureau estimates that 107 billion people have ever lived, which means that for every one person now alive, approximately fifteen people have died. There comes a tipping point in the timeline of our own lives when we know more of the dead than of the living. We all have forgotten much more than we remember. The proliferation of vanishing, more and more, is what we have to live with.

And yet disappearance does not necessarily mean obliteration. I hope that what remains might be enough, that beholding something as quotidian as a dead body's dirty laundry might be enough to ignite and kindle undying devotion.

For all of his losses in old age, I have come to feel that my grandfather—Jack *as Jack*—did not vanish. He persisted, a complex conglomeration of the past and his new present. Jack would mock-sing into a saltshaker when good music came on in the nursing home dining room. What else but an affinity for life was behind the enjoyment of playing instruments, traveling the world, perfecting omelets, and singing into a saltshaker? Stooping over his wife's coffin, deep in dementia, Jack said, "I don't want to join you yet, babe!" What else but a will to survive was behind piloting a cargo plane across the treacherous Burmese Hump, scraping his way through medical school playing gigs in bars at night, and declaring at my grandmother's graveside his desire to live? The essences behind his previous life endeavors seemed intact in Jack until the end—in subtle shades, often known only to those who spent time with him—while the activities that once embodied them had fallen away.

The mystics might say what is left is a truer, purer self. The dissolving of all doing, the stripping away of the *via activa*, makes straight the path for the naked, beloved self to emerge. The deconstruction of ego can facilitate a new freedom of being.

•

The definition of "vanishing point" seems to integrate apparent opposites. The point at which parallel lines receding from an observer converge at the horizon is also the point at which the lines disappear. The vanishing point is both unification and dissolution, the point of convergence and cessation.

If I stand still and watch a person walk away from me, she grows smaller and smaller, until she reaches the vanishing point. She has not vanished from the planet or from herself—she has vanished only from my view. If I move toward her, she reaches her vanishing point more slowly; if I move away from her, she reaches it sooner.

Kitwood argued that as the degree of neurological impairment increases, the person's need for psychosocial care increases. What traditionally happens is the exact opposite. As the degree of neurological impairment increases, the person becomes increasingly neglected and isolated, further increasing neurological impairment—a vicious circle. Malignant social psychology hastens the vanishing point. Person-centered care, which aims to affirm identity and promote well-being, tries to keep the vanishing point far off, to keep the person with dementia in view as a unified whole. The benefits of person-centered approaches, including the reduced usage of psychotropic medications among residents in long-term care settings, have been well documented. The Alzheimer's Association 2018 Dementia Care Practice Recommendations, a comprehensive guide to evidence-based quality care practices, names person-centered care as its underlying philosophy, pointing to research showing that individualized care decreases depression, agitation, loneliness, boredom, and helplessness among people with dementia, and reduces staff stress and burnout.

The vanishing at the vanishing point, however, is an illusion. A road does not cease at the horizon; it simply disappears from an observer's view. The person with dementia exists beyond my capacity to keep her in my line of sight; she remains a person despite my (or anyone else's) limited powers of vision. Still, we must reckon with the disappearing—even if it is, in some sense, illusory.

Leonardo's *Last Supper* contains perhaps the most famous vanishing point. Our eye is pulled into Christ's *head* at the center of the composition; it is the aggregating point. We are drawn to and through the mind of Christ—both to disappear there and to gather there. Christ dies on the cross (dissolution); Christ merges with the divine (unification). As we reach the vanishing point, we both dissolve and converge.

•

Having previously made arrangements with a Detroit funeral home for Janet Adkins's remains, her husband, Ron, headed straightaway to the airport to catch his flight back to Portland on the afternoon of Janet's death. "He wanted to get out of our jurisdiction as quickly as possible," one prosecutor involved in the case told the *Los Angeles Times*. "He wanted to disappear."

Ron Adkins publicly voiced support for his wife's decision, but I wonder if he pled with her not to do it—that it might be his honor to be burdened by her. Perhaps he resented his wife's determination that he should not be asked to do so. Perhaps he could come up with nothing more pressing in his life that would render caring for his wife a lesser good. Perhaps he was willing to risk their futures. He had purchased his wife a round-trip ticket, in case she changed her mind and wished to return to Oregon with him.

I have witnessed many loving partners unable to rise to the occasion—and perhaps this is what Janet Adkins wished to avoid. I have seen one spouse keep the other alive by any means necessary because the idea of being without the person was simply unbearable. Maybe Janet Adkins knew that love is blindness at times. Maybe the only person she trusted was herself, in the present—and a pathologist in Michigan.

I don't think Janet Adkins wanted to kill herself—rather, she wanted to kill her *future* self, the deteriorated self she imagined, the self she worried would put her family "through the agony of this terrible disease." The Janet Adkins on the tennis court and at the piano killed the projected Janet Adkins in a wheelchair, unable to find notes on an instrument whose name she cannot recall. The self-determining Janet Adkins killed the dependent Janet Adkins. The strong Janet Adkins killed the weak Janet Adkins, before the weak Janet Adkins got a foothold. The story is a familiar one: the strong subjecting the weak—the strong eradicating their fears through expulsion of the weak. Is this not the fascist impulse, the imperialist compulsion? Or might it be the compassionate impulse, the yearning to be free of unnecessary affliction? How blurry the distinction between exterminating weakness and alleviating suffering.

•

What does it mean to vanish well? After all, the result is always the same: you end up gone. There are no tricks to undo this finality. Magic's familiar script—the sudden deletion into thin air; the breathtaking reappearance out of thin air—does not seem to apply in the end. The stage assistant's role, however, may abide.

Perhaps, to vanish well entails allowing others to help unbind you, trusting them to keep your secrets. I think of Dorothy, who stood just offstage, offering a measure of knowing assurance, as Houdini attempted improbable escapes. We need compassionate attendants who help us in our final stages of disappearance, too. I think of my mother, soaking her dad's feet in a tub of warm water; of the nursing assistants, tenderly lifting spoons to open mouths; of Ron Adkins, sliding Janet's return ticket into his breast pocket. I imagine a world in which securing good support is not so hard, because living and dying with dementia is not so feared or fearful. For most of us, our vanishing will occur slowly and may mercifully give us time to gather willing assistants who know the illusoriness of disappearance when we reach the vanishing point.

3

Oh, Mexico

IN EARLY 2013, MY GRANDFATHER JACK MOVED TO THE Veterans Home in Mexico, Missouri. He was joining the ranks of the 1.4 million older adults who reside in nursing homes across the United States.

The facility was set on the edge of a remote town in the plains of north central Missouri. It was not an easy place to find. I had never been to that part of the state before Jack was moved there, and I doubt he had either. He would not get out of the car when he and my mother arrived. My mom had to walk away—racked with sadness and guilt, exhausted by the four-hour drive—while a nurse's aide coaxed him out. This was the third move he had made in three years; it would be his last.

My grandparents moved to Bonne Terre, Missouri, in 1953 after my grandfather had finished his medical residency. At the northern edge of the Ozarks, sixty miles south of St. Louis, Bonne Terre was a mining town, in a region known for having the richest lead ore in the world. During peak years of production in the early decades of the twentieth century, the mines employed thousands of people. A network of more than three hundred miles of underground haulage tracks brought the ore—a total of 8.5 million tons—to the surface. Once the profiteers exhausted the region's galena deposit—the largest in the world—they vacated the area. The Bonne Terre Mine closed in 1962. Within a decade, mining operations had ceased in St. Francois County and the surrounding area—what had constituted the Lead Belt—and had moved to the underexploited western side of the St. Francois Mountains, the *New* Lead Belt. After my mother finished college in the mid-'70s, she did not return to live in her depressed hometown. My parents settled in Cape Girardeau, about ninety miles southeast of Bonne Terre. Stretches of windy, two-lane highway with blind turns made the trip between them a particularly long, treacherous drive.

During one of my visits to Bonne Terre when I was in high school, my grandmother Edna showed me a painting on a dim wall in the guest bedroom. A farmer's wife had painted a pastoral scene of Bonne Terre's Big River and gave it to Jack for saving her husband's life. The farmer, who was half-blind, had picked up baby copperheads, mistaking them for big worms. That painting—its sparkling stream knifing through springtime bluffs, rolling along groves of weeping willows and fields of wildflowers—suggested resonance with the early French settlers' designation of the area as *la bonne terre*, "the good earth." The landscape of the town I knew was marked by littered highways, run-down trailer parks, and an eroding chat dump—a large mound of lead-flecked sand, left over from mining operations. I once scaled this chat dump with my cousins on a hot day during our summer vacation; my mom remembers sledding down it in the winters of her childhood.

In 1992, the EPA identified the Old Lead Belt as one of the nation's most contaminated areas, designating it a National Priorities List Superfund Site; it remains on the list. In 2003, the Eastern Reception, Diagnostic and Correctional Center—the facility where the state executes all its capital offenders—opened in Bonne Terre. This cluster of nineteen metal-roofed buildings, located on a barren 213 acres, inspires one to think neither of good nor of the earth.

After Edna's sudden death in 2009, my mom knew her dad could not live alone. He had trouble thinking and had relied on his wife to keep their household running. My mom left her job and home in Cape and moved in with her father in Bonne Terre, until she could figure out a more sustainable arrangement. Four months later, my mom moved Jack into an assisted living facility near Bonne Terre. He had lived in St. Francois County for nearly six decades; it was home to his church, beloved Rotary club, and former medical practice. It seemed worth a try to see if he could situate himself there.

Soon after the move, it became obvious that there was no compelling reason for him to remain local. The trip proved too far for my mother to drive regularly, which left her navigating, from a distance, new complications regarding Jack's care, such as his resistance to bathing. No one from Bonne Terre visited him anyway—no one from Rotary or the church—or, if they did, they did not communicate these visits to my mom. Within the year, my mom moved him to a memory care facility in Cape Girardeau, near my parents' house. Even if Cape had never been Jack's home, it had been home to his daughter and her four children—and our sense of place felt somewhat transferrable to him. Even though I had moved from Cape by the time he had relocated, I could still situate him there. *There* had history for me; I knew the borders, the landmarks, and the people.

Long before Jack's move to Cape, my parents had decided that eventually they would uproot to be near their most rooted kids—my two siblings who lived in Columbia, a town four hours northwest of Cape. They were in no rush to relocate, wishing to spare Jack another upheaval. However, through an unexpected series of events, my parents received an offer on their house, before it was for sale. With the housing market still tenuous after 2008, they accepted the offer. Two years after settling in Cape, Jack would need to be moved again.

Jack's new home was not to be in Columbia, however. He was moved forty miles northeast of Columbia into the Missouri Veterans Home in Mexico. He was a proud WWII veteran, and the facility was known for providing good, affordable care (and Jack liked nothing more than a good deal). A bed had just become available. These factors outweighed the fact that Mexico was a place distant from and unknown to my family, a place in which Jack likely had never set foot.

I had no stories of Mexico, Missouri—no memories in it, no mental or emotional anchors—which made Mexico hard to map onto the geography of my mind. It felt vacant, empty. In some ways, Mexico, Missouri, felt as distant to me as Mexico the country, also a place I had never visited. But I could at least conjure some images of the country, however partial, based on media depictions and the photos and stories my friends from Mexico had shared. I drew a total blank when it came to Missouri's Mexico.

I often had trouble remembering that Jack lived there. I had to remind myself he was there somewhere, in a little room, in a small town, in a part of the state unfamiliar to me. I could never remember how to get there exactly. Even though I regularly sent him cards, I always had to look up his address, his precise Mexico residence never imprinting upon my memory. He was not entirely gone from me as long as I could write to him, I thought. I imagined my notes, a row of triangles erected on his dresser, forming a little fence against isolation. I longed for attachment to the place, to him.

I saw Jack in Mexico only a few times. I lived in New Jersey and visited Missouri infrequently. The second to last time I visited him, I thought it would be the last. It was a beautiful fall afternoon. The floor nurse, who kept her little dog on a leash by the medication cart, told me Jack was still in bed. When I entered the room, he did not seem to register my presence. In the weeks prior to my visit, my mom had noticed his flat affect and increasing remoteness, but I had hoped I could inspire a different response. I had brought him M&M's, which had been his favorite, but he refused to open his mouth. I played big band music on a little CD player by his bed and held up old photos for him to see—all activities that had seemed to resonate with him in previous visits. He closed his eyes or stared straight ahead, his body motionless. I assumed he was tired of this world and ready to take his leave before too long, so I shut off the music and put the albums away. I sobbed quietly and said goodbye and prayed near his ear and kissed his head and had trouble walking out the door. It took the fifty-minute drive back to Columbia for my puffy, red face to lighten.

The last time I saw Jack was on Memorial Day weekend. I did not permit myself goodbyes or tears, now convinced that his fundamental hardiness would sustain him beyond all reasoning. This time, he was dressed and in the television room. It was another beautiful day. Flags lined the driveway up to the facility. I pushed his wheelchair outside on a concrete walking path and stopped at a bench with a small canopy for shade. I told him it was Memorial Day. I sat facing him and gestured toward the flags, but he peered past me to the magnificent pin oak in the open field. I told him I remembered the big trees in his yard in Bonne Terre and how he had dubbed his house "Oak Pointe" and had engraved a wooden OAK POINTE sign, affixing it to a tree at the end of his driveway. (How strangely domestic the French "e" had become in that most unpretentious region.) I told him he made incredible things out of oak, cherry, and walnut in his woodshed. I lightly touched his hand. He made no visible response to any of my overtures—the pin oak drew his whole attention. I stopped talking.

We had never before sat together in silence. When I was a child, he was forever in motion: playing his trombone for me, teaching me a new computer program, working in the yard. I was forever trying to find some entry point into his activity— some way to connect beyond his showing me something, making me something, teaching me something. Here we were now at rest—and I was squirming. I had trouble knowing what the stillness meant: *depression, apathy, serenity, emptiness, resentment, peace?* The small awning offered no cover; the relentless sun, coming at a late afternoon angle, struck us entirely.

When I brought Jack back inside, the nurse with the dog asked him if he had a headache. He made no motion. "Oh, yes, your head hurts. Here is some Tylenol." She gave him the pill and he took it. I wondered if she saw a response that I could not. I knelt beside him at the table, looking him in the eye. I did not know what to do or say, but I wanted a sweet sign—a smile or word from him I could report to my mother to make her feel better, to make myself feel better—to believe nothing was hurting. Instead, he narrowed his eyes and frowned. He scrunched his nose and forehead and shook his head, making a little mocking face back at me. This smirk was the first visible

reaction he had made to my presence during the visit—a retort
I read as possibly playful but mostly bitter, even sarcastic. *I don't
need your pity.* I took the sneer as a sign to leave. I gave him a
peck on the cheek, told him I loved him, and slipped out of his
view for the last time.

Here is one way I read our final visits: Jack was tired of
trying to find and refind his social footing, and was no longer trying. I don't mean he consciously decided to become
apathetic, but perhaps he sensed how difficult it was to relate
and how close failure was at every attempt. I think it became
easier, less painful and exhausting, to be docile. The speech pathologist Rosemary Lubinski notes that when individuals with
dementia "perceive that their responses are futile, they stop responding." Tom Kitwood makes a similar point, warning that
if the person's need for inclusion is not met, he or she "is likely
to decline and retreat, until life is lived almost entirely within
the bubble of isolation." By this view, Jack's withdrawal was not
due to his disease process alone. Rather, it was a response to an
entire social environment unable to support him.

It was not that Jack's caregivers were particularly negligent,
or that, had he been surrounded by more solicitous conversation partners, he would have been able to communicate profi-
ciently. But it seems that when little is expected from persons
with advanced dementia, little is given to or received from
them. The sneer Jack gave me was an expression of unnamable
anger—not so much with me personally, I like to think, but
with the forces that had brought him to this place of exile, a

bubble of isolation, cut off from anything and anyone who had ever signified even a semblance of *home*.

Mexico was the site of dislocation: Jack's final removal from his former life. In Mexico, he was not the man who stitched up bleeding heads and treated snakebites, nor was he the decorated pilot. Although he was surrounded by veterans, he no longer recalled his war stories—or, at least, no longer told them. He was not the jazz musician, or the Rotarian ambassador, or the philanthropic donor. He was Jack who didn't say much, who liked his morning coffee, and who sang on occasion. He was Jack with glowing skin and a full head of soft, white hair, who was a "Total Assist," requiring help with every daily activity from dressing to bathing. Once he had delivered babies, now he was diapered. Once he had traveled the world, now he shared a room, divided by a retractable curtain, with another slight, contracted man.

In this more pessimistic light, I saw Jack's successive moves, farther and farther away from anyone or anything familiar, as stripping him of any grounding in who or where he was. The insidious extraction of his life unfolded in sequence: his own home (fifty-seven years), assisted living near his hometown (nine months), assisted living near his daughter's home (two years), a nursing home in unknown Mexico (two years). He lived his final days in a place detached from any place he had known, cared for by strangers. His emotional distance should come as no surprise—what handle had he to grasp, what anchor served to hold his rocking vessel?

Each move was not intended to do any harm; inertia simply took over. While my grandfather may have had the financial resources to allow him to stay in his home by hiring round-the-clock caregivers, the prospect of relying on strangers to live with him in a semirural setting, with no close neighbors and my mother two hours away, would create a particularly vulnerable setup for him. Perhaps he could have lived with my parents. But they would have struggled to offer the continuous care my grandfather needed while managing their own lives. Not to mention that he and my grandmother had never so much as stayed overnight at our house when I was growing up, balking at the idea of "imposing" on my parents for even one night, let alone for an indefinite period. In the wake of my grandmother's unexpected death, coordinating Jack's care fell to my mom, who had some help from her sister who lived in Florida. Like most family caregivers, they did the best they could amid few viable alternatives.

I felt the weight of Jack's distance each time I took the spur off I-70 at Kingdom City and headed due north, past farm fields and blank plains sky, to an unfamiliar exit. I sang James Taylor's "Mexico"; the song's carefree scenario and wistful longing for the country of Mexico's sweet sun and bright moon soothed the sting I felt for my token visits to this remote place, to a man I had trouble locating. However, even Taylor's Mexico contains a reality check—a paradise lost—sad letters from home, financial ruin, hard times. Not even Mexico's hot sun and bright nights could protect against life's inevitable blows. And Jack's Mexico—the one in Missouri—was not a vacation destination, a make-everything-all-right utopia. Mexico, for him, spelled separation.

"Oh, Mexico!" I sang in full voice, windows down, my face toward the horizon's vanishing point. "I guess I'll have to go now!"

•

Jack's story, while personal for me, is not particularly unique: an old person, frail of mind or body or both, lives out his final years in a nursing institution, under the watch of paid staff, segregated from the wider community. Given that nearly a million and a half people in the United States live in nursing homes, institutionalization of elders is not a private, isolated phenomenon. There are nearly 16,000 nursing homes and another 30,000 assisted living facilities in America. Senior housing is big business. Long-term nursing care costs $6,844 per month, on average, for a semiprivate room. An average assisted living apartment costs $3,628 per month. Medicare covers neither. According to the CDC, 50.4 percent of residents in nursing homes have a diagnosis of Alzheimer's or some other form of dementia. As the ratio of adults under sixty-five to adults over sixty-five continues to drop, staffing these facilities will become increasingly difficult. Mexico is not Jack's problem or my family's problem alone—it is a public problem.

As I reflected on my grandfather's moves, as well as those endured by the residents I came to know in the Gardens, I began to question this arrangement—one that makes it so hard for so many old people to remain situated in their neighborhoods and communities, requiring them to exchange the rhythms of home for the regimentation of clinical care. At times, the ubiquity of elder care facilities can seem to me to be emblematic of malignant social psychology—a form of banishment and exclusion, physical or emotional.

"Banishment" in the context of care homes is often interpreted in narrow ways: disallowing a person to participate in a group activity, or placing a person in her room without access to others. At this micro level, I have no reason to believe Jack suffered banishment at the Veterans Home. However, from the vantage point of the larger movements of his life and the lives of others like him, I can't help but see the marks of banishment. In Jack's case, he was sent away from his home of fifty-seven years; he was sent away from the region he knew; he was excluded even from Columbia, the new epicenter of his daughter's family. He ended up on a landlocked island—physically out of sight and psychologically out of mind. He became a foreigner in the middle of his own home state. It is unlikely he knew his coordinates or could have located Mexico on a map. But my sense is that he possessed some awareness of being cut loose, adrift in no-man's-land—and his utterly subdued affect, I believe, may have had something to do with this awareness.

It is not that all nursing institutions are abysmal or that nothing of value can or does go on within them. They are often the only alternative elders have to languishing—physically, emotionally, spiritually—in their own homes or in the homes of overextended relatives, without the help they need. Perhaps the only thing worse than having nursing homes is not having them. It is what they represent that troubles me: the movement of frail old people to the fringes, out of common life, and into "the kingdom of the sick"—to borrow Sontag's illustrative phrase. They represent the readily available, readily agreed-upon societal solution to elder care, which involves relocation—more accurately, *dislocation*. That these institutions provide communities of care otherwise denied to elders, I can't help but feel, indicates a larger societal failure to welcome, integrate, and support them in neighborhoods and the greater community.

Like the insane asylums of the nineteenth century, might the presence of separate homes for elders in the United States reflect the prejudices of a dominant culture—a culture that finds institutionalization a viable remedy to the problems represented by certain populations?

The geriatrician Bill Thomas, a self-proclaimed nursing home "abolitionist," contends that traditional nursing homes represent the "declinist" view of aging—that is, the notion widely held in our society that older people are broken human beings who are less than they used to be. Rather than whole persons who continue to develop through their lifespan, old people are assumed to be in universal decline. This decline, so the declinist logic goes, rightly constitutes the elder's primary identity as "patient" and determines her living environment as increasingly estranged from normal life and ruled by medical

structures. Rejecting a declinist orientation, Thomas maintains that while growing old entails elements of decline, "the
larger truth is that aging is a complex, multifaceted, and poorly
understood component of *normal human development*."

While the facility where I served as a chaplain was well run,
the staff most often warm and caring, with an atmosphere of
community spirit often emerging among the residents, it was
ultimately still a clinical regime. I observed the residents anxiously line up (or, lined up) for their medication before each
meal; residents were interrupted no matter their present activity to be given their pills; residents had little privacy, ever under the watchful eye of the clinical imperative to prevent falls.
There were nurses' stations, medication carts, long corridors,
noisy common areas, and few small cozy spaces. Residents'
rooms had ceramic industrial-grade floors and harsh overhead
lighting. Floor staff wore scrubs. There were dining hours and
showering schedules. A four-digit code punched into a metal
keypad unlocked the doors of the dementia unit.

The events that precipitate this mass displacement of elders
from their homes are not highly visible communal catastrophes.
No disaster—no war, flooding, famine—initiates the everyday
expulsion of elders in modern America. The processes are
slower, more covert, and less openly violent than other forms of
banishment, and perhaps that accounts for why we have been
slow to name the injustice. Old persons in the United States

are not deported at the hands of conquering nation-states, but rather they are moved, more often than not, by loving caregivers. They are not going to places called Fort Lincoln Internment Camp or Willard Asylum for the Chronic Insane, but rather they move to places with names like Sunnyside Gardens or Seaside Manor.

The displaced population of elders, having internalized pervasive negativity about their own old age, often swallows their segregation as the proper and humble course of action. They know their place: step aside and do not be a burden. I have observed this many times in my work. Many elders—especially those, like my grandfather, with diminished mental powers—simply are not in a position to enact concerted, organized resistance, even if they wish to. I imagine a similar dynamic is encountered by those in our country who possess little power to self-advocate due to limited English skills, financial resources, and legal protections. They, too, know too well what it is to have someone else fasten their belt and lead them where they may not wish to go. Elder displacement, in a sense, is contiguous with the displacement (or threat of displacement) endemic to other vulnerable groups. Whether disabled of mind or body, poor or dark skinned, an ethnic or religious minority, exiles are rarely from the ranks of power and privilege.

New models are pushing back against the dominant setup, giving me some reason for hope. I had the good fortune of spending an afternoon at one of these alternatives. Memory Care at Allen Brook, in Williston, Vermont, had opened a few months before my visit in April 2018. It is a ranch-style home, where fourteen residents who have dementia live in individual apartments and share cozy, natural-light-filled common spaces. When I arrived, the smell of cookies baking in the kitchen wafted through the living room, where some residents were chatting and playing cards, while others were watching a nature film. I noticed that the telltale signs of a health-care institution were absent; there were no medication carts, no hospital floors, no long, sterile hallways. None of the staff wore scrubs or institutional name tags, making it hard to distinguish the residents from the employees and visitors, which I discovered was precisely the point. My tour guides, Ellen and Ken, the home's administrators, introduced me to each resident. "Lynn, this is my friend Dorothy. Dorothy, this is my new friend, Lynn." "Lynn, I'd like you to meet my friend John." The residents were called friends, not patients, not even residents. Ken explained, "We use the word 'friends,' because, quite simply, we *are* friends. Other language puts up barriers, making an 'us' and a 'them.' We don't want those kinds of barriers here. We want a real community." No sooner had Ken said this than a woman slammed down her playing cards and began to shout at the woman seated next to her. Conflict is part of real community, too, Ken added. He calmly approached the angry woman and invited her to go on a walk with him.

I learned that staff and volunteers were trained in the Best Friends approach to dementia care, a model that emphasizes developing positive, authentic relationships and respecting the basic rights of people with dementia, such as the right to be treated as an adult. But it did not seem the caregivers were rotely following a prescribed protocol—rather, a truly person-centered orientation, an abiding commitment to mutual well-being, had taken hold. "This is the first time I've had a job that didn't feel like a job," Ellen commented. "During my recent vacation, I literally couldn't wait to get back here and see everyone."

The Green House Project, founded by Bill Thomas, is another alternative model, in which elder care occurs in small, affordable, egalitarian homes for even the most mentally and physically compromised residents. Each house provides ten to twelve seniors with twenty-four-hour nursing care within a homey environment, with the intention of returning dignity and control to elders.

Other visionaries are focusing on the creation of dementia-inclusive neighborhoods. The Japanese gerontologist Emi Kiyota's Ibasho Cafés re-engage elders within their larger communities. These cafés, run by elders, are organic, informal gathering places for people in the surrounding community to find their *ibasho*—"a place where one can feel at home, and be oneself"—through intergenerational respect and sharing. The geriatrician Allen Power, in his book *Dementia Beyond Disease*, envisions an "Inclusive Society" in which models of

segregation, including most forms of dementia-specific housing, are abandoned in favor of solutions that "reintegrate those
elders into the fabric of the larger community." This involves
transforming personal values, redesigning neighborhoods, creating reciprocal, intergenerational networks, and educating
the general public about how to support neighbors living with
dementia.

Encountering these models offered me a window on what
might be possible. While new options seem to be slowly
spreading (there are 263 Green Houses in thirty-two states,
as of this writing), the supply of these kinds of revamped communities surely lags behind the demand; the home I visited in
Vermont, which admits only low-income residents, already had
fifty-three people on the waiting list. I do not believe there is
one answer. I am not searching for *the* "cure," but I have come
to see that there are more humane options. And part of finding solutions requires striking at the roots of the injustice, un-
earthing the forces behind displacement in the modern exile
of older adults.

The particular displacing mechanisms at work in senior
housing reveal, I believe, an especial American sin: our idola-
trous love affair with youth and the consequent obsession with
eradicating non-youth. The proliferation of all programs and
products *anti-aging* exposes the iniquity and issues forth ageism's
strongest imperative: remove signs of aging from the individual body and the body collective. In 2016, Americans spent
about $16 billion on cosmetic surgery and minimally invasive

procedures. And we may be exporting our obsession. The global market for "anti-aging" products and procedures is on the rise; according to Orbis Research, this market was worth $42.51 billion in 2018 and is estimated to reach $55.03 billion by 2023. It takes only a cursory glance at popular media to note the ubiquitous images of youth and the dearth of representation of elders, especially old people rendered as rounded characters. Older adults are made to disappear from the workplace, too; once unemployed, adults aged 55 to 64 face a higher likelihood of staying unemployed long-term. Research published by the Federal Reserve Bank of San Francisco in 2017 revealed that older job applicants uniformly receive lower callback rates for interviews, than similarly qualified younger applicants. For administrative assistant jobs, women aged 64 to 66 had a 47 percent lower callback rate than women aged 29 to 31.

Behind ageism lies deeply ingrained values that, I am convinced, are linked to our economy. My mind turns from Mexico back to Bonne Terre; the fate of the Lead Belt seems to point to a system that perpetuates displacement.

•

St. Joseph Lead Company, a firm based in New York, set up its first mining operation in 1864, in St. Francois County's village of Bonne Terre. While small-scale mining had been in operation in the area for decades before its arrival, the firm (known among locals as "St. Joe") introduced the deep-earth diamond drill, which made the extraction process far more profitable because of its capacity to reach rich deposits hundreds of feet underground. Bonne Terre reportedly grew from small numbers to a city of several thousand by the early twentieth century, largely due to the diamond drill and the establishment of an iron foundry and a railroad to process and ship the ore. The earth was both good and lucrative—the two descriptors nearly synonymous in the American imagination.

By the 1930s, St. Joe had become a monopoly, having gained control of all the smaller mining operations in the area. In 1972, having depleted local lead reserves, St. Joe shuttered its last mine in the Old Lead Belt. Knowing no other way to support itself, the region suffered decline similar to other 1970s de-industrialized communities, like those across the Rust Belt.

In 2015, forty-three years after St. Joe ceased operations in the Old Lead Belt, one-fifth of St. Francois County residents lived in poverty. Only 7 percent of Bonne Terre residents had a bachelor's degree or higher (the national average is 33 percent), and nearly 16 percent of residents under sixty-five years old did not have health insurance, almost double the national average. In 2018, the EPA reported that, in the three zip codes that encompass the Old Lead Belt, between 9.3 and 16.7 percent of children had elevated blood lead levels; the national average is 2.5 percent.

St. Joe created local dependency on its jobs and, predictably, did not remain committed to the place and its people beyond their immediate use-value. This is, of course, often the industrial ethos: when profit can be maximized, workers and their land are quickly exploited; they are quickly discarded when the project is exhausted. The small history of the Old Lead Belt points to a larger history of elite economic interests overriding the local, long-term well-being of the individual and collective body.

I see this same dynamic, these same values, reflected in the ageism that underwrites elder displacement. In the industrialist framework, the body is imagined as machinery; it is only as good as its capacity to produce *like a machine*. Machines don't mature; they either work or they get replaced by ones that do. Old bodies are merely worn-out machines that possess suboptimal parts. They are past their prime, on the decline, sliding down to uselessness. If they have not already, elders join the ranks of others pushed aside by market values—the poor and developmentally disabled, for instance. Thrown off the line, discarded, and replaced. When what is profitable is good, and what is good is profitable, then persons who no longer produce—including the most rudimentary "goods," like coherent thoughts and sentences—are in danger of abandonment.

And as with old-model machines, when old bodies become obsolete, we have a disposal problem. There are so many old machines and such limited landfill space. There are so many old people and such limited space in our private and public lives. By 2030, older people will outnumber children for the first time in U.S. history; one in every five residents will be of retirement age. If older people have become no longer relevant to the machinations of modern life, we face the question: *Where do we put them?*

The farmer and writer Wendell Berry warns that an economy consumed by the immediate and obvious use of something, whose worth is judged by its monetary value, marginalizes the young and the old, who "are living either before or after the time of their social utility." Berry writes, "Any organism that is not contributing obviously and directly to the workings of the economy is now endangered." I read Berry's observation against the backdrop of my grandfather's repeated moves. Berry's critique hit close to home for me and resonated with my growing understanding of the connections among declinism, ageism, elder displacement, and the framework of our economy. The frail body, like the population of a town whose natural resources have been depleted, is now in danger of neglect, abandonment, and forced relocation.

In this schema, aging and the increased need for assistance are problems to manage and resolve, and the growing percentage of the population over sixty-five is an impending natural disaster (a "silver tsunami") that imperils the nation. But a less fatalistic approach is possible. If we shift our thinking and readjust our economy, we can begin to encounter and support old age as a normal, multifaceted aspect of life. If we are not old already, most of us hope to survive into old age. This rather basic impulse—not to die young—should offer some motive to consider the ramifications of our present order and the impermanence of our social utility.

•

On April 19, 2013, in Mexico, Missouri, in the dayroom on the skilled nursing floor where he had moved just a few weeks before, Dr. Jack Mullen celebrated his ninetieth birthday. I was told the card I sent him was pinned up on the door to his new room, where his twin bed sat to the right of the retractable curtain. I have no idea whether or not anyone read the card to him, or if they assumed he wouldn't understand anyway. My mom sent me a video. Jack is in his wheelchair, clapping, as the small gathering of family sings "Happy Birthday." His youngest great-granddaughter waves a red pom-pom. His oldest daughter is taking a picture. His sons-in-law look strained in their singing and clapping. On the table beside Jack sits a gift bag, a small cake, and a half gallon of 2% milk.

On this same day, 1,030 miles from Mexico, in Princeton, New Jersey, in 1879 Hall—the building of Woodrow Wilson's office when he served as the university's president before becoming *the* president—I watched my spouse defend his 470-page dissertation in a conference room full of the most elite scholars in his field. We clapped when the chair of his committee pronounced him *"Dr.* Ryan Harper." We raised our flutes of champagne and toasted to him in the 1879 Hall lounge, where we nibbled on cheese and crackers, miniature pastries, and fruit. There was laughter and hugs and palpable relief at the completion of such a passage. I sent a proud email that evening to my friends: "Ryan successfully (and, if I may say, quite brilliantly!) defended his dissertation this morning!"

I was applauding an intellectual feat, among some of the best minds in the world, in a bucolic university town, nestled in the center of power, halfway between New York City and Philadelphia, in the shadow of presidents and future presidents. Jack was applauding and being applauded, at a remove from the center of anything, in the shadow of monocultures and ethanol refineries, unable to speak his children's names, unable to play his instruments, unable to control his bowels. I applauded scholastic achievement; they applauded sheer survival, the inexplicable persistence in the midst of long-standing brain disease. This dispatch from Mexico reminded me that we never know when our circumstances will change, when we might swap one form of applause for another, or exchange a mahogany-appointed lecture hall for a linoleum-floored multifunction room.

•

Rather than only a site of dislocation, perhaps Mexico was a place where Jack could find welcome relief, where he could, as James Taylor's song suggests, lose his load and leave his mind behind.

In Mexico, Jack bonded with Linda, a retired nurse hired by my mom to visit him several times a week. A Mexico local, Linda was a foreigner to my family and me. Since she did not know Jack before his move into the facility, Linda was free to be with him just as he was. He didn't have to work to maintain a former identity, or play a former role, or keep a story line intact. For the first time since his wife's death, Jack had a companion who was there for him consistently. A companion who, for the first time in a decade, was not involved directly in assisting him with hygiene, meals, or medication. No wonder he perked up when he saw her. They sat together, sipping McDonald's coffee, slowly bringing in the new day.

To build a life in exile, one must draw more upon inner states than outer forms. Many of the exiled ancient Israelites came to understand the precepts of their faith as somehow lodged within them, written upon their hearts—not located in a particular city and its temple. The mystics of faith affirm this wisdom. A fourteenth-century guide to contemplation, *The Cloud of Unknowing*, whose writer succeeded in remaining anonymous, says, "Nowhere, physically, is everywhere spiritually. Understand this clearly: your spiritual work is not located in any particular place." Viewed from this angle, Mexico could be the site of freedom—a monastery, a retreat, a hideaway where Jack could live without the judgment of others who held him in and to a different time. The freedom of a physical nowhere, a placelessness, could make way for spiritual ubiquity—to *be* finally, with abandon. Since he no longer had to (or could) maintain the various masks of white, middle-class manhood, perhaps he could relax into himself at last, with a new companion who understood him as he was. Mexico, a nowhere place, became uniquely his—a place I located only through him, a place only through which I could locate him. Neither withering in the long shadow of his former self nor subsumed in his daughter's new Columbia life, he could reside in a new land, *his* land, a kind of pure land.

I don't believe that displacement is holy, that people who are displaced should give thanks for the spiritual opportunity. But I have begun to hope, lately, that spiritual work—what I see as the yearning for and the mysterious manifestation of love, meaning, and purpose—can at least persist in the midst of exile. Jack had never seemed poor in spirit or meek; I never sensed a trace of self-doubt in him, never saw him shrink from the spotlight, not even in the early years of his dementia. He had loved the attractions of life and drank deeply from life's various cups, but the time of indulgence was over, and the path had turned spare and arid. In his final years, humility seemed near to him. One way I could read his flat affect, I suppose, was as hallowedness—that he had touched a new place within himself, meek and mild, free from what is assertive, controlled, and strong. He was inheriting the earth; he was losing his life only to find it; his was the kingdom of heaven. Not in a saccharine or triumphal way, not that his struggle reduced to a spiritual lesson he had to learn. I simply hold on to the hope that his secret heart knew a certain secret happiness.

There is no one story that puts all the pieces in place; no

one border that can be drawn and guarded that contains the total of his Mexico, or that contains the wide and sprawling territories of any life. Borders are crossed; boundaries move. We keep searching for them, creating them, relocating them. And with each step we take we uncover a contour, a plain, a valley, a hill that we had not noticed or recognized or named before.

One legendary account says that Mexico, Missouri, got its name by a certain convenience of signage. L. Mitchell White, editor of the *Mexico Ledger* in the 1960s—while admitting that his history might be shaky—reported that the town's first settlers found a wooden sign along the trail. The marker pointed southwest, and on it had been painted MEXICO. The settlers figured that rather than replace the sign, they might as well call their town Mexico.

I initially balked at what seemed like the settlers' lack of originality and self-respect in such haphazard naming, but perhaps they simply took the practical and humble course. At its inception, Mexico assumed itself to be a passageway to somewhere else—a place that points in the direction of another place, like a finger pointing to the moon. And because of Jack, Mexico became somewhere to me, pointing me to him and to the swaying pin oak that held his attention in the field on our last visit, to light and solitude and the recesses of a placeless home.

•

His body arrived in Bonne Terre from Mexico two days before the funeral. He was buried on a bitter cold, gray afternoon, three days before Christmas, in a cemetery across the street from the chat dump. The graveside service fell to me. I began with Job: "I know that my Redeemer lives, and that in the end he will stand upon the earth." An old man from the VFW, dragging his bad leg, approached the coffin and offered a veteran's prayer. Two baby-faced privates folded the flag and presented it to Jack's children.

I felt the tightening of my throat, stopped to feel my breath, before I offered the committal. *Ashes to ashes, dust to dust.* I stood still, stiff from the merciless cold and grief. I hesitated to move from the plot. There was no other place to go. He had returned to the good earth, to nowhere and everywhere.

4

Turning to Fools and Madmen

As I plumbed the dimensions of dementia and the sources of its particular dread, my earliest memories of encountering mental disability—memories that had all but vanished—began to surface. They involve Diana, a girl who lived down the street from my family when I was a child. Seemingly out of nowhere, Diana would show up in our garage. Sometimes she would make it through the garage and into the kitchen. Her desperate moans, her high-pitched pleading voice, often gave her away before we saw her imposing frame. She had grown large during early puberty, but her thin, stick-straight white-blond hair had not changed. Her hybridity confounded me: she possessed the body of a full-grown woman and the fine hair and reasoning capacity of a toddler. No longer wearing her leg braces (perhaps they did not fit after her growth spurt), she walked with a limp, and she walked fast when she was determined. She would tear down our driveway, blowing past my dad, who was hunched over machine parts in the garage, and enter our house. From the bedroom or living room, my mom, siblings, and I would hear her heavy steps and raspy wail in the kitchen. We all knew what her presence meant: Diana had run away again.

I was friends for a time with Diana's older sister Tracey, in the way you become friends in elementary school: largely based on grade level and geographical proximity. We roller-skated to music in her driveway, choreographing our favorite routine to Paula Abdul's "Straight Up (Now Tell Me)." On the rare occasions when we played inside, I recall her house as dark—the windows draped with heavy curtains—and the walkout basement smelling of cat urine. I have few memories of Tracey coming to my house. In retrospect, I can see that she had to stay close to home to help out with Diana—or to keep an eye on her baby brother, while her mother tended to Diana.

Diana's soft features appeared unusually stretched. Maybe a fraction of a centimeter, maybe the length of a mustard seed or two, separated her facial proportions from kids who weren't called "retarded." It's the word we used for Diana, meaning no particular offense. At the time, my siblings and I knew that she was not like us, and that we should never mock her (my parents made that clear). But I now cringe at my use of such an insensitive term, which reduced her to her difference from us. Tracey once pulled out an album and showed me her sister's baby pictures. Diana had tubes taped to her red face; even then, her face looked too broad. Tracey did not say a word about the reason for the tubes or why she wanted to show me Diana's birth photos, why I needed to see her troubling origins. It seemed as natural to her as roller-skating to Paula Abdul tapes.

I am not sure, even now, why Diana would run away to my family's house in particular. We lived on the same street as Diana's family, but on the other end, a quarter mile or so from their house. Diana passed by many houses similar to ours, each plot nearly identical to the next, before she descended on our split-level. Her mother—a heavy woman with dark, deep rings under her eyes—would often arrive a few minutes behind Diana, huffing, in hot pursuit. After her growth spurt, Diana stood a head taller than her mother, who was not short herself. Now, with little physical leverage over her daughter, Diana's mother seemed even more exhausted, her eyes even more depressed. We looked down and waved off her apologies when she appeared at our house to fetch Diana, which was perhaps our Midwestern way of protecting Diana's mother (and ourselves) from embarrassment, as she goaded her daughter out of our house and back down the street.

I did not know what Diana wanted with those visits; I never thought to ask her. Although I had witnessed her grow red in the face, shake her head fiercely, tears and snot flinging from

her face, I never saw Diana turn violent, and to my knowledge she had never harmed anyone. We said we were scared
for Diana—scared for her to get hit by a car, scared for her to
get lost, scared for her to get taken, scared for her to get scared.
*Poor thing. She just doesn't know where she is. She gets so upset. She's so
big now. So hard to manage.* While she often appeared distressed,
I wonder now if we failed to understand the true nature of
her expressions, dismissing them, out of hand, as irrational, as
unavoidable "agitation."

When she showed up at our house, I think we felt nervous—
not just nervous for her, but nervous for ourselves, about nothing we could define clearly. Madness seemed to intrude upon
us, stalking us—showing up, wailing, in our family's driveway,
garage, kitchen—a displaced yet known entity. Diana's unpredictable interjections into our lives felt unsettling, disrupting, even threatening. These impressions spoke to a deep and
complex discomfort, internalized early, associated with mental difference. I have since noticed a similar nervousness that
permeates, at times, interactions with people who have dementia; I am curious about this correspondence.

•

In 1901, Auguste Deter was admitted to the Hospital for the
Mentally Ill and Epileptics—known colloquially as the *Irrenschloss,* "Castle of the Insane"—in Frankfurt, Germany. Her husband did not know what else to do with his fifty-one-year-old

wife, who had apparently gone out of her mind. Her psychia-
trist, Dr. Alois Alzheimer, studied her and kept careful notes.
On November 29, 1901, four days after the patient's arrival,
Alzheimer recorded in her medical chart:

> During physical examination she cooperates
> and is not anxious. She suddenly says, *Just
> now a child called, is he there?* She hears him call-
> ing [...] When she was brought from the iso-
> lation room to the bed she became agitated,
> screamed, was non-cooperative; showed great
> fear and repeated, *I will not be cut. I do not cut
> myself.*

Earlier in the examination, when she was unable to complete
a writing task Alzheimer asked of her, she repeated the phrase
I have lost myself. In Dr. Alzheimer's 1907 article "On an Unusual Illness of the Cerebral Cortex," published a year after
Auguste's death, he writes:

> The first symptom the 51-year-old woman
> showed was the idea that she was jealous of
> her husband. Soon she developed a rapid loss
> of memory. She was disoriented in her home,
> carried things from one place to another and
> hid them, sometimes she thought somebody
> was trying to kill her and started to cry loudly.

Shortly after Auguste's death, Alzheimer, who was by then a researcher at the Royal Psychiatric Clinic in Munich, requested her file and had her brain sent to him. From slides of her brain tissue, he observed peculiar clumps of abnormal proteins and dense bundles of neurofibrils in the cortex. These beta-amyloid plaques and neurofibrillary tangles, whose exact role in the disease remains uncertain, are believed to block communication between nerve cells and contribute to their death. The patient whom Dr. Alzheimer called "Auguste D" became the first person identified with the new brain disease. It was named after her diagnostician. The most common dementia-related disease was delivered in and to the halls of madness. It was as a psychiatric patient in the Castle of the Insane that Auguste Deter became Alzheimer's first named victim.

Alzheimer's disease, originally referred to as presenile dementia, was a rare diagnosis in the first decades after its discovery, because it applied only to people, like Auguste, whose dementia occurred before age sixty-five. Older people with the same symptoms were not given the diagnosis, under the assumption that their cognitive decline was simply normal for advanced age. This distinction dissolved in the late 1970s. The historian Jesse Ballenger's 2017 article "Framing Confusion: Dementia, Society, and History" explains this evolution. Through the work of a coalition of caregivers, family members, researchers, and government officials, the categories of senile dementia and Alzheimer's presenile dementia were combined into a single entity: Alzheimer's disease—and thus became a major public health issue, contending for federal dollars. "Campaigns organized around this reframing of dementia were highly successful," writes Ballenger. "By 1980, Alzheimer's had become a household word and the object of a massive federally funded research initiative." Despite these extensive research efforts, now spanning over four decades, Alzheimer's disease remains poorly understood. The FDA has approved only two types of drugs—cholinesterase inhibitors and memantine—to treat the cognitive symptoms of Alzheimer's disease; neither type stops the disease's progression.

The National Institutes of Health defines dementia as "the loss of cognitive functioning—thinking, remembering, and reasoning—and behavioral abilities to such an extent that it interferes with a person's daily life and activities." A set of symptoms, dementia is caused by a number of different conditions, including degenerative neurological diseases (such as Alzheimer's and Parkinson's), vascular disorders that impede blood flow in the brain, traumatic brain injuries, and certain types of infections. Alzheimer's disease, the predominant cause of dementia, accounts for 60 to 80 percent of cases. Of course, dementia has not always been so clearly or narrowly defined. Before dementia became regarded as the product of disease in the twentieth century, it was a broad concept associated with insanity and applied to those who exhibited psychosocial incapacity, disorganized behavior, or diminished ability to reason. In the decades following Dr. Alzheimer's discovery, the age-associated dementia we now know was steadily disentangled from this catch-all category. Nevertheless, through the first half of the twentieth century, old people with dementia who were unable to live in their communities still were often linked to insanity and committed to state mental hospitals. They became one of the largest segments of the patient population.

Dementia's etymology—*de* (out of) *mentia* (the mind)—reflects roots in madness. And the extent of madness's stigma is vividly, if grotesquely, reflected in the treatments used upon people deemed out of their minds. Foucault's classic *History of Madness*, and the sociologist Andrew Scull's contemporary work on madness, elucidate this long and unsavory history. In premodern Europe, madmen were often bound in chains, kept in cold, dank cells, and subjected to all manner of cruelty in the hope of exorcising insanity's source. Purported to be possessed by evil powers, the madman was deemed to be overflowing with invading spirits, legions of them. After overtly religious explanations and cures were abandoned, practices of sanctifying madmen endured in the form of medical procedures and moral censure. Common medical treatments of the seventeenth and eighteenth centuries included immersing maniacs in ice water, using blood transfusions as a remedy for melancholia, having madmen ingest soap and tartar, and soaking patients in vinegar. Some reformers of those eras made a turn toward moral approaches; they utilized what became known as the "silent treatment," including the use of solitary confinement, to urge sufferers toward a state of reflection and (they hoped) self-correction. In the nineteenth century, new technology promised new routes to healing. A rotary device rapidly spun patients, who were strapped in a suspended chair, often to the point of nausea and incontinence, as a means to restore their mind-body equilibrium. Benjamin Rush, a signer of the Declaration of Independence who is sometimes called the father of American psychiatry, created a special "tranquilizing chair" designed for sensory deprivation. He also recommended bleeding and purging patients, and the ingestion of mercury.

In the twentieth century, pharmacological interventions rose to prominence. By 2013, one in six Americans—and one in four older adults—reported taking a psychiatric drug, according to data gathered by the Medical Expenditure Panel Survey. And while these drugs are a far cry from bloodletting and ice-water baths, their side effects can be severe, ranging from emotional numbness and suicidal ideation to sexual impotence and metabolic disorders. As I mentioned previously, the risky, off-label use of psychotropic drugs with people who have dementia is common as a means of managing certain behavioral and psychological symptoms of dementia (BPSD), such as anxiety, agitation, and depression. Some person-centered care activists, such as Allen Power, reject the category of BPSD. Viewing people through the lens of BPSD, asserts Power, "causes us to medicalize and pathologize the expressions of people living with dementia." While some people with dementia may legitimately need medication to treat a mental illness such as depression, Power maintains that these drugs too often are administered under a misguided notion that they are necessary to quell signs of distress. Rather than address the source of people's distress and holistically support their well-being, we resort to dangerous chemical interventions.

The long-standing cultural impulse to segregate and suppress people who are cognitively different may account for some of dementia's present-day stigma. Of course, we now understand dementia as the product of disease, not a form of madness, and, thankfully, have abandoned the cruelties of, say, spinning chairs and sensory-deprivation therapies. Nevertheless, the taint of madness persists—and may explain some of dementia's dread. Dementia activates our deep-seated fears of "going insane," Kitwood posits, because it confronts us with the terrifying prospect of "unbeing," of the corrosion of one's sense of self. This largely unconscious dread might explain (at least in part) the highly defensive ways in which we often respond to people with dementia. Left buried and unaddressed, these fears generate negative patterns of relating to these people—Kitwood's "malignant social psychology"—which, he warns, functions to "exclude those who have dementia from the world of persons," and which at times might accelerate their mental decline.

But what particularly about "going insane" engenders fear and malignancy toward people who represent mental instability? Some clues may lie in how conceptions of madness function to stigmatize the mad. According to the sociologist Erving Goffman, once stigmatized, a person is reduced "from a whole and usual person to a tainted, discounted one"—and thus is readily excluded from the world of persons. The madman, says

Foucault, "crosses the frontiers of bourgeois order" and "alienates himself outside the sacred limits of its ethic." He acquires stigma, becomes tainted and discounted, through his incompatibility with "bourgeois order"—that is, white, upwardly mobile social norms. He is irreformably inefficient and entirely unmarketable.

No matter its source, madness is trespass, an unauthorized border-crossing from the land of prudent productivity into the land of reckless idleness. Those who have transgressed—those who have "lost their minds" from birth (Diana) or sometime after (Auguste)—violate the sacred limits of industrial order, which narrowly calculates human value by our capacity for mechanistic production and conspicuous consumption. Unable to maintain respectability in this schematic, lacking both efficiency and potency, the mentally disordered are punished by the order they unwittingly defy.

Persons with dementia have *acquired* a cognitive disability, my friends in disability circles sometimes remind me. They become initiated into the stigma that others, who were born with brain impairments, have suffered their entire lives. All those whose brains are considered damaged or otherwise abnormal endure a similar process of outcasting, it seems—a social response that demands scrutiny.

Perhaps especially as a surviving incarnation of "madness," dementia haunts us with the specter of helplessness, irretrievable social demotion, and indelible stigma. Dementia threatens the myth that personal hard work and ingenuity can overcome all obstacles. While some fatal diseases can be ennobling, bravely battled or stoically accepted—leaving respectability untouched or even bolstered—Alzheimer's and other dementia-related diseases, in the popular imagination, spell unmitigated tragedy. Even when we know more about the pathology of brain disease, and even when we claim to be beyond assigning moral meanings to illness and disability, dementia remains a special case of violation. It is not only physically and mentally debilitating but also socially devastating.

Elderly persons with dementia are at risk for what sociologists call "social death"—a condition in which people are treated, for all practical purposes, as if they are nonexistent. In their 1997 landmark study on dementia and social death, the psychologists Mary Gilhooly and Helen Sweeting observed that the determining factors for social death often coalesce in people with dementia: advanced age, lengthy fatal illness, and loss of personhood (commonly linked to the ability to recognize others). One-third of the family caregivers they interviewed not only expressed the belief that the continued existence of their relatives with dementia was pointless but also treated those relatives as if they were socially dead. The woman who kept her husband on the back patio in the cold of winter, the man who strapped his wife to the toilet while he left the house to run errands, these caregivers regarded their loved ones as, in some significant sense, already gone. These extreme cases highlight the threat of depersonalization for people living with dementia. Older persons with dementia are at greater risk of mistreatment than those of the general elderly population; the National Council on Aging reports that nearly half of elders with dementia have suffered some form of abuse. The notion that persons are "already gone" surely contributes to such high levels of abuse and neglect. The subtler, more common intimations of social death—the many small ways in which we steer clear of people with dementia—underscore the same stigma.

I recall visiting a church that had asked me to speak about ministry to people with dementia. The leader of the congregation's pastoral visitation group told me that, while my material would be helpful for the visitors, she would *never* assign them to visit someone with severe dementia. A pastor friend confessed to me that he does not visit a longtime member of his congregation because the member's son tells him not to bother, saying his mother "wouldn't remember anyway."

Within the walls of the CCRC where I worked, I witnessed a pecking order emerge in which residents with severe dementia fell to the bottom of the heap. Residents who volunteered to visit their frailer neighbors in the Gardens often specifically asked me *not* to assign them to the dementia floor. These peer visitors wished to spend time with people who were "with it" enough to "appreciate the visit." (I came to understand that "appreciate" usually meant "recall the visit later.") In all of the above cases, the visitors in question are those who offer their time and energy to the work of compassion, whose ethic compels them to care for vulnerable others. Even among them, a prejudice cuts deeply against persons with dementia. And it's

not just them. I have noticed how my own reluctance has sur-
faced at times, and how my own feet have dragged.

If the fear of "going insane" lies beneath the fear of dementia,
if part of dementia's stigma stems from the shame surrounding madness—then we would expect *madness* to still find its way
into dementia descriptors. Given madness's close association
with dementia's etymology, history, and special threats, we
might expect the images swirling around dementia to gravitate,
still, in twenty-first-century America, toward lunacy, if they
gravitate toward anything. Seldom, however, do I hear people
with dementia referred to as "insane" or "crazy" these days—or,
strangely enough, even as "demented."

Perhaps, we have overcome this particular misconcep-
tion. Now, it seems, we know at least a little better—or, more
truthfully, we know a little *more*. Brain scans, lab tests, mental exams, genetic testing, and medical histories help physicians determine diagnoses. But if I had lived at the turn of
the century, and if my wife hid objects around the house and
screamed loudly about someone wanting to kill her, I would
have suspected she had gone mad, too. I would have grown
frightened and admitted her to the nearest *Irrenschloss*. Now we
have mostly disassociated mental illnesses and dementias from
"insanity," mercifully abandoning the moralistic categories
and remedies of bygone eras. We discriminate among different
forms and sources of psychological distress. We better grasp

the physiology and distinctive features of different illnesses. We know not all persons with cognitive abnormalities require the same sorts of treatments and services. We know that people can have both dementia and mental illness, but the conditions are not synonymous. People can have dementia with or without psychosis. We have moved away from labeling people, whatever their mental state, as "crazy," "insane," or "mad." Equipped with newer and better information, we fancy ourselves free from premodern prejudices against people with damaged brains. We know they are not mad—they are diseased.

If we believe Susan Sontag's claim, that as scientific knowledge about a disease increases, fear-driven images and moral judgments about its sufferers dissipate, then we should rightly expect metaphors around brain disease to die, too. Might madness and its attending metaphors, with all their moral and spiritual baggage, be casualties of enlightenment—and, if so, should we expect that prejudice against people with dementia is going to steadily die?

Perhaps. But the shedding of prejudice rarely comes so simply and reasonably. The dearth of madness-speak might signal progress—or, at least, would not seem so conspicuous—if we took a similarly wary stance toward other dementia metaphors. I suspect, however, that our fear has not so much abated as it has attached itself to a different set of images, in particular the images of absence. Allusions to the progressive nonexistence of people who have dementia seem to crop up in nearly every corner of dementia discourse.

A 2010 *Time* magazine cover brandished the word "Alzheimer's" in large, bold letters across a woman's half-faded head; from crown to neck, she is only half present. A 2008 Alzheimer's Association advertisement showed a washed out, phantasmic older man in a tuxedo holding the arm of his daughter in a wedding dress; another ad in this series showed a similarly ghostlike woman at the dinner table with her granddaughter, who is holding a newborn. When a prominent journalist interviewed the University of North Carolina's legendary men's basketball coach Dean Smith in 2014, the year before Smith's dementia-related death, he described Smith as a "ghost in clothes" with "empty stares." Another reporter described him as "alive but absent." My friend's words about my own grandfather often revisit me: *Oh, so he's gone.*

Rather than one condition among others, dementia takes on apocalyptic overtones of annihilation. Brain disease evokes the removal of the person in ways other progressive illnesses do not. Images of half-gone or faded persons do not typically accompany, say, heart or liver disease. A person dying of lung cancer is not a ghost in clothes. Dementia, these depictions suggest, never adds to or leaves equal—it only subtracts from the person *as a person.*

The rhetoric of vacancy, in our century, triumphs over lunacy. It seems we favor the mind *in absentia* as opposed to *in dementia.* The person is not crazy; she is simply gone. Favoring the dissolution of persons over their disordering may seem, on the surface, a more humane gesture. "Mom is fading" sounds less ugly than "Mom is batty." To be sure, there are good reasons to divorce dementia and other brain-altering conditions from madness, but I fear the move to vacancy, rather than mitigating dementia's stigma, may actually intensify it. For starters, oblivion metaphors seem not to square with actual experience. I know what the *actual* brain-dead look like, although I wish I did not know. I have seen vacancy.

The worst job I ever had was as the on-call chaplain for an organ donation network. I carried around a pager, night and day, dreading the call. In order to be eligible to donate one's vital organs, the donor candidate typically dies from traumatic head injury, and is pronounced brain-dead. One case I worked involved a man who fell off his bicycle and hit his head. Another case I recall was a man who tried to hang himself, whose girlfriend found him suspended from a cord in his garage. Both men had no blood flow to their brains. Their pupils were fixed and dilated. All reflexes were gone, even the breath reflex. These patients looked as flaccid as corpses, except for the modern peculiarity that their lungs continued to rise and fall and their hearts continued to pump—wholly by machine assistance, until the moment right before the removal of the organs.

I found the job unbearably gruesome and sad. After working a few cases, I tendered my resignation. I knew there was hope on the other end for the organ recipients and even hope down the line for the devastated families I encountered. My

orientation to the job had been replete with heart-melting tes-
timonies of generosity and gratitude. However, I was not on
that other end. I was on the fixed-pupils end, the weeping end,
the found-my-lover-swinging-from-the-rafters end.

Brain death, in my experience, does not resemble dementia, even advanced dementia. A palpable life force abides in
persons with dementia—sometimes a discomforting life,
but a life to encounter, engage, and know nonetheless. They
make motion and express emotions; they act and attempt to
act. Personal expressions endure, however subtly. Their highly
symbolic language requires sensitive interpreters and compels
creative response. And at their dying breaths, I have witnessed
their entire bodies release and cease, coming to an organic rest.
They were never still-breathing casualties, like the brain-dead.
I have never encountered a person with advanced dementia
as appearing even *virtually* brain-dead; they must be reckoned
with as individuals with distinct ways of being in the world. In
fact, of the two, lunacy more than vacancy would better describe certain encounters I had with people on the dementia
unit in the Gardens.

I recall Pearl, who could shake the building with her
screams, and Lena, who sang songs from her days in the Hitler
Youth, claiming the facility piped these jingles into her apartment. Barbara would slam her walker against the dining room
wall, and when she saw me in her rage, she implored, "Pray
'Our Father' for me." Freda, a retired kindergarten teacher,
saw schoolchildren in her room in the middle of the night and

taught them their classroom lessons. Joe sang at the top of his lungs when no music was playing. It is hard to construe any of these residents as gone—rather they appeared more disordered than empty. Their expressions ring more of mental disturbance than mental absence, and speak to an *abiding* self (albeit a distressed self, at times) rather than to an *absent* self.

This "virtually brain-dead" ideology, this absenting of persons with dementia, relieves caregivers of both anxiety and responsibility, says Kitwood. It allows the psychological barriers to remain high. Even in care settings marked by greater flexibility and lower psychological defenses, Kitwood notes, "[t]he anxieties surrounding dementia are very great, and the unconscious is highly ingenious in creating new forms of avoidance." More than a third of people living with dementia reported losing friends after they received a dementia diagnosis, according to a 2013 report by the UK's Alzheimer's Society. This fact seems to point to the anxieties surrounding dementia, which result in avoidance of persons with a diagnosis. While descriptions of dementia patients as brain-dead represent the far extreme of vacancy metaphors, any intimation that a person is gone alleviates culpability. I have little responsibility for the well-being of someone who is actually *no one*. When one's mind has vanished rather than warped, if it is gone, then our guilt can recede. We are relieved of the pressure of having to relate to a person with a mind still there but deformed.

While there is a troubling moralism attached to lunacy, there is an equally troubling nihilism attached to vacancy. The former cloaks dementia and its sufferers in spiritual judgments; the latter purges dementia and its sufferers of meaning or of any potential for meaningful existence. Attempting to neutralize our fears of going insane, we vacate the mind from the body—*the light's on but nobody's home.* It seems we have simply replaced the superstitious *filling* of the person with demons, with a superstitious *emptying* of the person of intention and meaning. *She is not aware; he does not know; his stares are empty; she does not recognize, just a ghost in clothes.* How are these claims anything but metaphysical?

To be sure, certain cognitive capabilities—language and motor skills, types of recall and spatial processing—diminish with dementia, but when we pronounce another human *absent, gone, empty, unaware,* we assume that we have a kind of godlike knowledge. Awareness—that complex constellation of intellectual, emotional, somatic, spiritual *knowing*—is irreducible to my and others' limited perceptions. Subjected to highly circumscribed scrutiny of their cognition, persons with dementia often receive labels that tell only partial truths about their capacities and can feed the myth of absence.

The neuropsychologist Steven Sabat's 2001 book *The Experience of Alzheimer's Disease: Life Through a Tangled Veil,* a seminal work among person-centered-care advocates, highlights the subjective experience of people living with dementia. Through his interviews with adult daycare participants, Sabat notes the emotional complexity of his subjects' experiences for which mental exams failed to properly account. One interviewee, a retired academic and scientist, had scored poorly on mental exams, and his Alzheimer's disease was termed "moderate to severe." By standard metrics, he possessed little or no cognitive ability, yet he eagerly participated in Sabat's research—what the participant called "the Project," "a sort of scientific thing," that brought "*real* stature to do." Sabat discovered that the tests used to assess the interviewee's cognitive abilities "did not tap his need, nor his ability, to maintain feelings of self-worth," which remained intact. A particular assessment tool had pronounced the man "gone," but had not accounted for the whole picture of someone who craved recognition as a highly educated person who longed to contribute to a worthy project.

I recall Vera, a resident on the dementia unit, whom the floor staff had told me did not speak or interact with others— she was "disengaged" from her social environment, they said, due to her severe cognitive impairments. In what turned out to be her final months, Vera attended the unit's weekly interfaith spirituality group—the small gathering that Vera's late evangelical neighbor Betty had helped form. Far from disengaged, Vera always appeared alert and intent, making eye contact with me and other group members. If we gave her ample time, she would offer a word or two to the discussion. When the group learned that she loved cats, we began to incorporate feline-themed pictures and poems into our meetings, which made Vera smile. I remember her son's shock when he visited from out of town and found his mother participating in the group.

Auguste Deter, Dr. Alzheimer's patient, supposedly

exhibited "psychosocial incompetence," which was one definition of dementia at the time. But I have read Dr. Alzheimer's
interviews with her, and I do not find Auguste incompetent. I
find a person pregnant with psychosocial longing, with desire.
As she repeats her name, *Auguste, Auguste*, I hear her sensitivity
to her own person and the threats to her personhood. When
she repeats, *so anxious, so anxious*, as the doctor questions her, I
sense an emotional awareness; she knows something is amiss.
When Alzheimer asks her on what street she lives, Auguste
answers, *Well, this is Frankfurt am Main*, revealing her perception
of her general place. Her anguished, *I have lost myself*, reveals her
abiding sense of self ("I"/"myself") and her feelings of grief
during her examination. When she was brought from the isolation room to the bed, she "became agitated, screamed, was
non-cooperative; showed great fear and repeated *I will not be cut.
I do not cut myself*." I can think of no more appropriate response
than terrific fear of bodily and psychological violence, given
she had been kept in "the isolation room" only to emerge in a
strange place to a probing male stranger.

In the midst of Auguste's mental deficiencies, many of her
expressions, the feelings behind them, make good emotional
and psychosocial sense, yet the doctor sees them as defective,
just another manifestation of his disease. The treatment of
Auguste Deter evidences a clinical, distant, depersonalizing
approach to dementia. It centralizes mental tests that make
little account for symbolic language, the motions of the body,
or the intimations of desire—tests that fail to examine how the

examiner impacts the patient's response. She is an empty person, a patient only, a peculiar case of brain disease, devoid of psychosocial competence.

Auguste Deter died on April 8, 1906, at age fifty-five from blood poisoning due to an infected bedsore—"lying in bed in a fetal position completely pathetic, incontinent," reports Alzheimer in his 1907 article.

I understand the comfort that may abide in the notion of vacuity, in *absenting* the diseased person, as a gesture toward compassion. I did not want my grandfather, or any of the residents in the Gardens, to suffer as their conditions progressed. If personhood is gone in the late stages of dementia, then they are spared any grief that may come from an awareness of both their own dying and the anguish of those around them. Given the unknowns of the subjective experiences of persons with severe dementia, I see the consolation in imagining blankness for them—especially if the alternative is torment. If we envision the person as either moving toward emptiness or anguish, vacancy will win out every time as the more humane vision. But too often we confine individuals with dementia to these two options, reducing persons in all their intricacies in order to fit them into this schema. The geography of the inner world defies such orderly mapping; we flatten the soul's contours when we persist in imagining only polarities.

A vision of vacancy, a death before death, may offer solace

to individual caregivers, but in the end, it serves to oversim-
plify dementia experiences and to remove people from full
moral accounting, which has troubling connections to other
historic injustices. Drawing upon her experience as an African
American, Lela Knox Shanks, in her 1996 memoir about caregiving for her husband, Hughes, resists the notion he is anything but fully human throughout his dementia. "One reason
slavery endured for so long in America was that some propo-
nents promoted the idea that the Africans had no souls," she
writes. "It is a dangerous and degenerate society that engages
in the dehumanization of any segment of its population." But
if the mind has not left but has changed, morphed into something unsettling and unpredictable, then we must make our
response. We can cover the dead—or those presumed to be
gone—in a nostalgic haze, talk of them in the past tense. The
"mad" must be regarded in the undomesticated present.

What if we defied vacancy's tyranny and returned to madness for a moment—not as demon possession or constraint
or a way to classify and contain people—but as needful folly
in a world of stifling convention? Vacancy seems to suppress
imagination; madness stirs it. Might we direct these motions
toward compassion? Madness, understood as a window on a
social world less ruled by mental conformity, might have some
salvageable meanings for dementia. Metaphors, our enduring need for enchantment, do not evaporate in the cool fluo-
rescence of sound information. Resistant to obliteration, our
symbols require reconsideration; they need both pruning and

flourish. So I want to explore the wreck—to plumb madness's metaphorical world for redemptive possibilities.

If we let it, madness might just purify us: upsetting our narrow order, recovering the latent wisdom in our folly, and restoring us to foolishness. The "mad," the "insane," the "demented," the "disabled"—they unsettle us, the temporarily able, with their bald truth. And we need unsettling, if we are ever to be anything but semiconscious sleepers, virtually brain-dead to the world. We need to be saved from our own vapidity, from our own diminished spirits and vacant imaginations.

King Lear's Fool, a prime representative of madness's reordering, punctures the pretenses of wealth and power, exposing the frailty that lies behind human facades. In a fit of petty rage and poor judgment, Lear recklessly disowns one of his daughters, the loyal Cordelia. His other daughters, the conniving Regan and Goneril, cast out their father after he gives them their inheritance. Lear's kingdom, his political and familial power, his mental and physical prowess, are all slipping away. Anguished by his loss of stature and identity, Lear pleads, "Does anyone here know me? [. . .] Who is it that can tell me who I am?" Despondent, the old monarch refuses to seek shelter during a violent storm. As rain pelts his head and thunder and lightning hem him in, he taunts the tempest, inviting its wrath: "Rage, blow! [. . .] Vaunt-couriers of oak-cleaving thunderbolts, / Singe my white head." Lear, however, is not alone in this storm. The Fool stands beside him, and perhaps it is he who knows Lear and can tell him who he is.

Refusing to abandon the king in his fit of suicidal rage, the Fool tries to convince him to go inside: "O Nuncle, court holy-water in a dry house is better than this rain water out o' door." Given his own small stature and humble estate, the Fool is uniquely positioned to accept Lear in his folly, in his new stripped state. As Lear descends further into despair, the Fool abides.

In a moment of affection for the Fool—and perhaps with a faint but growing recognition of his own folly—Lear says, "The art of our necessities is strong, / That can make vile things precious [. . .] Poor Fool and knave, I have one part in my heart / That's sorry yet for thee." The Fool and the chastened king, for once, share a common lowly condition. And in this state, "vile things" (such as the Fool) become precious to Lear. He values the Fool in a new way, not for what the Fool can do for him but for his loyal companionship. "He that has and a little tiny wit," sings the Fool, "Must make content with his fortunes fit, / Though the rain it raineth every day." Lear pronounces the Fool's jingle "true." This affirmation provides a window into Lear's growing solidarity with those of small estate and perpetual misfortune, those of "tiny wit" for whom "it raineth every day." Lear, too, must learn contentment with such small "fortunes." Lear's Fool says only a few lines, appears infrequently, never receives a name beyond Fool, and exits the play cryptically and abruptly—to kill himself, some scholars speculate. Obsolescence, it seems, marks the vocation of such fools. It is little wonder that the Fool is especially equipped to accept the bitter and broken king, that he alone bears witness to the Lear who confesses, "I fear I am not in my perfect mind."

In light of cognitive impairment, the Apostle Paul's declaration—"God chose what is foolish in the world to shame the wise"—becomes concrete. By the Apostle's logic, fools are not incidental to the holy; they are not reluctantly included in the kingdom; they are not welcomed as an act of charity on behalf of the rest of the community. Rather, they are chosen. They are *choice*. They are choice as opposed to castoff; choice as opposed to burden; choice as opposed to no one important or, more to the point, as simply *no one*. Given a seat of honor, not a cup of bitterness. Paul's choice foolishness is marked by humility, offering nothing to the world but one's lowly estate. At the mercy of others, these fools possess no special power or privileges, finding companionship and meaning where others see only waste, or nothing at all. In this regard, "fool" is not a slanderous term, but rather it indicates a kind of blessedness. Lear's Fool, by this definition, is no vile thing.

Mary, one of the residents I came to know at the Gardens, comes to mind as a "fool" in the positive Pauline sense, too. Her acute anxiety, on top of memory issues, made getting out of bed a herculean task each morning. When she finally did, she would often set to work, helping her neighbors in wheelchairs get to activities and meals. Some days, Mary shook too violently to speak. I could often tell the emotional tenor of

Mary's day by the accuracy of her lipstick application: the more the color strayed from her lips, the more anxious she was. She made a point to come to the weekly spirituality group I facilitated on the dementia unit (sometimes she transported Vera in her wheelchair). One day, we reflected on the Beatitudes by reading a contemporary rewriting of this series of blessings from the Sermon on the Mount. The first line said, "Blessed are you when you don't have it all together." Mary, a crooked red line extending past her lips and halfway down her chin, immediately chimed in, "I must REALLY be blessed then!" She had the group in stitches. She keeps disarming me.

In one of the first books on the spiritual needs of persons with dementia, *A Guide to the Spiritual Dimension of Care for People with Alzheimer's Disease and Related Dementia: More than Body, Brain and Breath*, Eileen Shamy also appeals to the value of foolishness. A Methodist clergywoman, Shamy declares in the introduction that she hopes the book will bring together those who work with and love people who have dementia. She describes this communion as a "fellowship of the foolish." "For foolish we most certainly will appear," she writes, "in a society obsessed by the quantifiable, by the immediate, by productivity and usefulness, by competition and profit, by individualism and loss of community, and where the bottom line really is the bottom line." In such a world, Shamy asserts, "it is accounted madness to expend precious resources on those who in economic terms are useless." It is a scandalous fellowship, this fellowship of fools, whose upside-down logic ordains the mad-minded, the weak-bodied, and the poor-spirited as bearers of divine wisdom.

During my chaplaincy training, I learned about the Reverend Anton Boisen, who, in the early twentieth century, found himself thrust into the "fellowship of the foolish." Boisen enjoyed a rather ordinary, if peripatetic, early career in ministry. He did survey work for the Presbyterian Board of Home Missions, served two short-term pastorates, and worked as the Congregational chaplain at Iowa State University. During World War I, he worked two years for the YMCA in France. None of these positions, however, represented Boisen's greatest contribution. His career took an extraordinary turn only after the pastor became the psychiatric patient.

Boisen suffered five major periods of psychosis, what he called "mental disturbances." During one of these episodes, his family had him committed to Westborough State Hospital in Massachusetts, where he remained for fifteen months. His diagnosis was dementia praecox, what we now call schizophrenia. Boisen recalled the one time a psychiatrist agreed to speak with him. The doctor's pithy response—"Nature must have its way"—disheartened Boisen, who felt the psychiatrist had missed the spiritual depth and intricacies of his condition. The disappointed Boisen realized the physician "had neither understanding nor interest in the religious aspects of my problem."

The ministers who came to offer Sunday services for the

patients at Westborough proved equally unhelpful. While they may have known something about religion, Boisen observed, "they certainly knew nothing about our problems." One minister preached a series of sermons on the state of missionary activity in Africa and Asia. Another pastor preached on the text "If thine eye offend thee, pluck it out." Boisen reflected, "I was afraid that one or two of my fellow patients might be inclined to take that injunction literally." The patients' spiritual hungers were systematically misunderstood or denied.

Boisen, however, listened to his fellow madmen and heard spiritual hunger; he listened to his own soul and heard a divine echo in its ache. Writing from the confines of his hospital ward in 1921, Boisen responded to a friend's suggestion that he could recover only if he gave himself over to "simple manual work": "Hang the sanity! You can't ever make life worth living if all you're doing is to try to keep from going insane." Who can blame the friend, who wished Boisen to busy himself with menial tasks in order to stay safely sane? The advice aimed to keep Boisen firmly away from foolishness, to keep his life small, ineffectual, faithless.

After his recovery at Westborough, Boisen committed his work and study to better understanding and serving those "who have been forced off the beaten path of common sense and have traveled through the little-known wilderness of the inner life." Reflecting on his new vocation, Boisen wrote, "I am not afraid. I have always managed to find my way through; and I do think that in a very real sense I have been exploring some little-known territory which I should like now to have a chance to map out."

With the help of his friend Dr. Richard Cabot, a well-known physician who taught social ethics at seminaries in Boston, Boisen became the chaplain at Worcester State Hospital and began to bring seminary students inside psychiatric hospitals for a supervised experience with patients, similar to the kind of practicum required of medical students. He wanted future ministers to encounter patients in all their complexity and potential, within the clinical setting, and he wanted the patients to have their religious lives, that "little-known wilderness of the inner life," taken seriously. These seminary students were adept at studying the Bible and theological writings, but Boisen felt passionately that ministers needed to learn to read a different kind of text—what he termed the "living human document." They especially needed to learn to appreciate the themes, metaphors, and movements of the inner life.

Boisen's experiment took hold, evolving into a transcontinental training program called Clinical Pastoral Education (CPE). I first heard of Boisen and his "living human document" during the first week of my first unit of CPE training, the summer I was assigned to the neurological unit. CPE, or some variation of it, is now a fixture in seminary curricula. Most major hospitals rely on CPE students and supervisors to provide spiritual care, and many denominations require their candidates for ordination to have at least some CPE training. An extensive board certification process for health-care chaplains, which many hospitals require of their hires, entails the completion of CPE units. Boisen's program has moved beyond his original focus on psychiatric facilities, expanding into nearly every clinical environment.

Origins, nonetheless, matter. Reflecting on Boisen's legacy, the theologian Robert Dykstra wrote in 2005, "Pastoral theology was born of madness and, one could argue, has yet to fully recover." When Boisen first began asking hospitals to allow in seminary students, he received pushback from skeptical hospital administrators. One superintendent, however, agreed to Boisen's proposal, saying he would let a "horse doctor" in if he thought it might help the patients. Ministers readily took their place alongside the horse doctor and the insane in the fellowship of the foolish.

Perhaps recovery is not the goal. The Catholic priest and writer Henri Nouwen says a Christian leader is called "to be completely irrelevant and to stand in this world with nothing to offer but his or her own vulnerable self." In a world full of peers who do things—or at least seem to do important things—to offer nothing but one's vulnerable self rings ridiculous. (What exactly does a chaplain, a minister, a writer *do* anyway?) By Nouwen's definition, it seems, Christian leaders cast their lot with people who find themselves—through no choice of their own—made insignificant, dwelling among the obscure, steeped in the fellowship of the foolish. The irrelevance, this foolishness, is not borne of naïveté or ineptitude. It is not the irrelevance of a preacher updating chapel-goers at a mental institution about global missions. It is the irrelevance of losing your life in order to find it; of loving madly without condition; of not having it all together. I now understand why I came to like working with people who have dementia. It is not because their pain is my pleasure; their suffering is not merely "interesting" to my otherwise boring life. Rather, all pretense ceases; their open dependency lays bare my less visible need for others, for help. Admitting my own limits strikes me as a gentler and more honest approach to life.

In every age, it seems, we want madness—however we define it at the time—to shut up, to turn vacant, to put on some clothes; we want to neutralize its danger and muzzle its unsettling truth. Boisen observed that "the real evil in mental disorder is not to be found in the conflict but in the sense of isolation and estrangement." I can't help but think of our propensity to isolate and estrange persons with dementia. While we do not literally consign them to life in an asylum, they do tend to reside on the fringes of our families, congregations, neighborhoods, and nation, and on the fringes of public discourse. We need healing. We must look again at the ones we have handed over to the margins.

On his way out west to do church surveys, as he passed through North Dakota, Boisen noticed from the window of his train "a large group of buildings standing in sharp relief against the horizon." He asked the man seated next to him what the buildings were, only to learn that he was looking at the state insane asylum. "I thanked him and thought no more about it," Boisen wrote. "It did not occur to me that I ought to be interested in those buildings or in the problem which they represent." Less than a year later, Boisen found himself "plunged as a patient within the confines of just such an institution."

I consider that passing train, the pale face in the window squinting at the distance. And how often I have been a passerby to someone else's bondage, a cool distance, catching a glimpse of something foreign on the horizon, something not mine, never to be mine. I see it; like all voyeurs, I am curious, but I do not see myself in it—or, at least, not yet.

Lear's Fool seems to understand how close chaos is to any one of us, how fragile are our own estates. "This cold night will turn us all to fools and madmen," the Fool famously declares. "This cold night" is a condition beyond human control—one among countless other circumstances that lie outside our power. Any one of them could turn any one of us into fools and madmen. The Fool states the case even more emphatically: the night *will* turn us, not *could* turn us. And it will not turn some— it will turn *all*. The Fool speaks a discomforting truth. Chaos will come to us all. Everyone is vulnerable; no one is exempt. When I have dementia. Never *if*.

5

The Golden Hour

IN CENTRAL NEW JERSEY, JUST OUTSIDE TRENTON, SITS Grounds for Sculpture, a world-renowned forty-two-acre sculpture park. Among other pieces, three-dimensional replicas of Impressionist and Post-Impressionist paintings populate the grounds. The local artist Seward Johnson reimagined Renoirs, Monets, Caillebottes, and Manets as life-size sculptures; visitors can walk among the figures, stand under the figures' umbrellas in a Paris rain, clink glasses with them at a boat party.

I arrived at this magical place for the first time in the fall, close to sunset. Through a narrow passage, I entered *Erotica Tropicallis*, Johnson's tableau of Henri Rousseau's *The Dream*.

Enclosed by a dense thicket of bamboo, the scene simulates twilight slumber. On a small couch lounges a pink-skinned nude surrounded by two lions, an orange snake, blooming jungle flowers, ferns, an elephant in silhouette, a citrus tree, tropical birds, and a snake charmer holding a horn to his mouth. The problematic colonial dimensions of Rousseau's 1910 piece—the fascination with "exotic" African themes and the portrayal of African subjects as primitive objects—occur to me now. It is telling that the dark-skinned man recedes into the backdrop among the other jungle creatures, while the light-skinned woman dominates the foreground. And it is perhaps equally telling that the male artist depicts a naked woman, and that no figure in the painting mirrors the artist's physical form. But, at the time, I was entranced by the magic realism of Johnson's representation, especially its play of light and dark.

Only the thinnest strands of evening light penetrated the bamboo cover, barely illuminating *Erotica Tropicallis*. Visitors stepped onto a small platform to insert themselves into the dreamscape—a good photo op if not for the prohibitively low light. I could not resist entering the scene, slipping in beside the slight man with the horn and just above the supine woman with her broad, perky breasts and long, streaming hair. I stood in a tight spot between the dark jungle and the light woman.

Grounds for Sculpture's description says the woman is "apparently oblivious to the danger posed by the wild creatures in her midst." Seeing her up close, I noticed her serenity, her half-smile—no tense lines, no tight muscles, at peace in her

dark dream and round body. Surrounded by shadowy creatures, obscured by the jungle's dense nightfall, languidly, she
reclines: naked, open, restful. She appears unafraid; she seeks
no escape from this dark kingdom, finding herself irrepressibly
there. Perhaps she is less oblivious than brave, less clueless than
wildly composed in the face of danger. Or maybe she understands that darkness does not necessarily equal danger. The
menace of the dark jungle may be, after all, a mere projection
of European anxieties.

I exited the scene, but it stays with me. Like the woman, I
long to lie in threats and deflect their power. I am practicing
repose, putting on a half-smile, and relaxing into falling light.
Like the figures in the shadowy background, I want to be at
home in lush obscurity. Lately, I am particularly interested in
whether gaining comfort with darkness might hold some potential for how we deal with dementia, and with the various
perils that come with aging.

•

At my grandfather's funeral, people apologized for my loss,
and if anyone had the courage to refer to my grandfather's
long-standing dementia, they mentioned the "dimming" of his
final years. In my uncle's eulogy, he spoke of his father's "dimming mind," and perhaps his words gave other funeral-goers
the acceptable lexicon to refer to Jack's last decade with dementia. At the time, the descriptor troubled me. I recalled

Susan Sontag's warning: "Disease metaphors are never innocent." I have become aware of how they often serve to stigmatize sufferers, adding layers of shame to illness. And how
dementia teems with fraught metaphors. I saw references to
my grandfather's "dimming" as another euphemism for progressive forgetfulness. The language was meant to be delicate,
yet it was related to a host of other damaging metaphors that
besiege persons with dementia. He was *dimming*, just like he
was *fading away, losing his mind, losing himself, disappearing in plain
sight.* This rendering, I thought, was a permutation on popular
zombie tropes, which imagine the body of someone with deep
dementia as "still going" even as the "real" person is gone. The
person slides into universal darkness, descending ever deeper
into a kind of unreachable obscurity.

After his funeral, the darkness of dementia—this metaphor
I was quick to rally against—would not depart from me. I began to stumble into it everywhere: in newspapers and maga-
zines, on television, in conversation. Alzheimer's "turns off the
lights" in the brain; it is "spreading darkness"; a "dark fog." It
is an "invading kudzu vine," blocking out the light. It "dims"
one's "fire." The eyes of sufferers are "void of light." To find a
cure, researchers must "decode the darkness." Once stricken
with the disease, sufferers steadily go dark, as their loved ones
"watch the lights go out." A reviewer of the 2014 documentary *First Cousin Once Removed*, which chronicles the poet Edwin
Honig's final years with Alzheimer's disease, describes Honig's
plight as "the steady dying of an intellectual light." The 2007

sequel to *Losing My Mind*, Thomas DeBaggio's popular memoir on living with Alzheimer's, is titled *When It Gets Dark*.

Darkness. It elicits its own special dread. In the moral imagination, darkness is synonymous with evil and menace, with sinister deeds hatched in the dark hearts of dark men. And in the intellectual imagination, darkness is equated with stupidity, empty-headedness. Someone who is *dim*-witted, according to Merriam-Webster, is "not mentally bright." In popular Christian spiritual imagination, darkness is associated with sin. Believers are children of light, lifted out of darkness— that place of great weeping and gnashing of teeth. They are the light of the world. Light shone in the darkness, and the darkness did not overcome it. The annual stewardship campaign of a church I once attended brandished the theme "Be the light, light the way." How warped we would deem the slogan "Be the dark, darken the way."

In common understanding, light triumphs, or *should* triumph, over darkness. The light/dark dualism has lodged itself in our individual and collective psyches. Disparagement of the dark, over the goodness of light, seems merely automatic—so embedded is the hierarchy in our lexicon. The association of darkness with dementia, whose derision also seems automatic, comes as little surprise. If enlightenment signals high moral, intellectual, and spiritual development, then endarkenment signals an inferior state in all respects. In this framework, dementia—envisioned as a darkening force—diminishes the moral, intellectual, and spiritual standing of its sufferers.

The historian Jesse Ballenger's *Self, Senility, and Alzheimer's Disease in Modern America* helped me better understand how such negative metaphors have become so endemic to dementia. In the late 1970s, in order for the newly formed National Institute on Aging (NIA) to receive levels of funding comparable to those of other institutes within the National Institutes of Health, the NIA needed a signature disease. Robert Butler, the first director of the NIA, pushed for a primary emphasis on Alzheimer's medical research—as opposed to broader foci on caregiving concerns and a variety of brain impairments, which many groups argued should take priority. Butler contended that biomedical research on specific diseases—highlighting their tragic, death-dealing aspects—was easier to sell to Congress than basic research. What Butler called the "health politics of anguish" buttressed funding efforts: the more horrendous the particular disease, the more urgent the need for finding a cure. Starting in the late 1970s, advocates worked to legitimize the need for Alzheimer's funding by stressing its singular devastation as not one disease among many but as the "disease of the century," the "most dreaded disease." While a host of negative metaphors emerged, the title of a 1983 seminal governmental report on living with Alzheimer's—"Endless Night, Endless Mourning"—appealed specifically to darkness to heighten anxiety and urgency.

A greater sensitivity, I believe, now exists among major health organizations around the use of certain stigmatizing language. Nevertheless, the overwhelming focus on finding the cure can still feed stigma. The first goal of the U.S. National Plan to Address Alzheimer's Disease, an outgrowth of President Obama's 2011 National Alzheimer's Project Act, is to prevent and effectively treat Alzheimer's disease by 2025. Campaigns like the Alzheimer Association's search for "the first survivor of Alzheimer's," while a provocative concept, render invisible those persons who are living long and well with dementia, suggesting that only those who are fully cured are considered to be survivors. The Pure Imagination Project, launched in 2017, uses images of a disappearing landscape to illustrate the effects of Alzheimer's disease, with the tagline: "Alzheimer's can steal your imagination piece by piece. But with your help, imagine how we can end it." The ad reinforces the idea that Alzheimer's causes people—or, at least, vital aspects of who they are—to steadily vanish, and that this thief must be stopped (cured). While, of course, the disease entails diminishment, these fundraising efforts often eclipse the many non-biomedical initiatives that are promoting the well-being of people living with dementia. They shift attention away from the examination of social and political factors, such as poverty and racism, which may contribute to high rates of dementia among certain groups; African Americans, for instance, develop Alzheimer's disease at about twice the rate of their white counterparts. And they also ignore the ways in which persons with Alzheimer's disease and their care partners do not always or only experience inexorable loss. A disproportionate emphasis on cures often comes at the price of promoting, however unintentionally, stereotypes and stigma around Alzheimer's "victims." Some dementia experts, wary of these tactics and the promise of a "magic pill," are approaching dementia differently. The neurologist Peter Whitehouse, author of *The Myth of Alzheimer's*, eschews the Alzheimer's diagnosis, seeing Alzheimer's as a spectrum of disorders rather than one disease that has *a* cure. The best tools for preventing and minimizing symptoms of cognitive impairment, argues Whitehouse, include public health initiatives around diet, exercise, and reducing head injuries and exposure to environmental toxins. He also stresses the importance of elders engaging in purposeful work, ongoing learning, and intergenerational relationships.

Although the narrative has shifted some in recent years, since the 1970s, Alzheimer's has been framed, more often than not, as a foreboding force that can be thwarted, ameliorated, and ultimately cured only through biotechnological advances—a logic predicated on what Ballenger calls "medical triumphalism," in which modern medicine is cast as the only or best source of hope. This disproportionate faith in medical science to solve all forms of diminishment, perhaps especially cognitive diminishment, persists. And I can't help but see the light/dark dichotomy at play in medical triumphalism: the light of medical technology will triumph over the dark of dementia; enlightened minds will save endarkened ones. In the meantime, the rest of us must simply watch while our loved ones "succumb to the darkness." Taking their place among other fear-laced dementia descriptors, the dark images swirling around dementia serve to deepen dementia's dread. They tap into our deeply embedded cultural bias against darkness, laying bare our dark fears and exploiting them to amplify the threat of Alzheimer's. It occurs to me that these images are a permutation on pervasive vanishing metaphors—darkness, after all, renders one invisible—but they carry an additional charge of stupidity, depravity, and menace.

However, in order for darkness metaphors to work in reinforcing an atmosphere of acute anxiety around dementia, we must continue to agree, however tacitly, to the premise that darkness is bad, wrong, fearful. This reflexive bias *for* light and *against* dark is in no way innocent. It splits the world into stark hierarchies in which dark and light exist not as two distinctive yet interdependent elements—each equally needing the other—but as disparate, opposing forces. Light-dark asymmetry both reflects and generates injustice (the history of racism bears this out in horrifying specificity). This dysfunctional division underlies the deception that light can (or should) exist apart from shadow, that the former rightly crowds out the latter—that boundless light signals boundless good. Such disunion maligns darkness and disavows its wisdom.

Are there ways to retrain our reflexive disdain for darkness and reclaim the dark's necessities and possibilities? How can we rehabilitate our implicit loathing for dementia and its so-called dimming? I don't have all the answers to this, but I believe that thinking about these issues—reflecting on them seriously, and with empathy—is the only effective way to move

toward a sense of balance. I suppose this book is a way of attempting corrections: to undermine light's supremacy, to affirm dark's worth, and to find a way of approaching dementia
that does not rely on such easy metaphors and polarities.

After my grandfather's funeral in 2014, I began the work of
trying to reclaim darkness metaphors. My pursuit led me to a
rather obscure figure from my past—to Father James, the only
Catholic professor at my divinity school. He was both brother
and father: a Benedictine monk and an ordained priest. Every
day he wore gray sweatpants and a logo-less gray hooded sweat-
shirt. His hands were regularly buried in his front pouch, fin-
gering his rosary. He had a greasy, unstudied comb-over, and
I don't recall him ever smiling. When I saw him in the gym,
he always held a small, ragged Latin prayer book to his face,
sweating and praying while he walked on the treadmill—never
noticing (or at least never responding to) my greetings.

Although I experienced Father James as terribly dour,
I did respect his commitment to a simple life of prayer and
modest means. While the teachings of other, more affable and
accessible professors entirely escape me now, bits of James's
premodern-inflected wisdom have returned to me in the decade since I finished divinity school. He claimed, without
apology or hint of irony, that the invention of the electric lightbulb is the source of much evil. It initiated a pivotal tide-shift
when we turned our back on prayer, scriptural memorization,

and the holiness of natural rhythms. My initial reaction to his assertion was utter dismissal. The capacity to light the night not only felt necessary and natural but also unquestionably good. What did a cranky monk, nose buried in the Latin Psalter, know about the way the world worked anyway? Now, as I increasingly distrust the assumption that light is always right, I revisit his theory for its shades of truth.

Our national sleep shortage may help prove Father James's point. Nearly one-third of adults in the United States do not get enough sleep, a fact the CDC calls an "unmet public health problem." Insufficient sleep precipitates an increase in motor vehicle crashes, industrial accidents, and chronic diseases. Constant artificial illumination (*be the light; light the way!*) contributes to our sleep epidemic. Because the light emanating from electric devices activates the brain and disrupts circadian rhythms, the National Sleep Foundation recommends a bedtime routine "conducted away from bright lights." The CDC names "round-the-clock access to technology" as a probable contributing factor to our dangerous lack of sleep.

To no small effect, excessive artificial light also creates the peculiarly modern phenomenon of light pollution, which simultaneously washes out the night sky and wastes energy. Most of us must travel long distances to see what our ancestors readily observed, pondered, and revered: the splendors of our own galaxy. Not only does artificial illumination directly and immediately disturb sleep and obstruct stargazing, it fosters a culture of constant stimulation and its diffuse damages. The growing darkness at day's end no longer dictates that we, too, must wind down. Rather, we plug in, flip on, and amp up. We never have to "power down" when we have ample electricity and ample machines to run on it. We can work ourselves, others, and the land, without end, it seems. We need not look up.

Perhaps debating the particular merits or deficits of the lightbulb is beside the point. Surely, we can count the ways the electric bulb has helped our lives, as well as the ways evil thrived *before* the electric bulb, too. The proliferation of light, without respect for darkness, signals a larger movement: the ceaseless escalation of human mastery over the earth. When we disallow darkness its regular place in our lives and permit light to rule the day *and the night*, we welcome imbalance. We tempt ourselves to more and more work and activity and, ironically, to more passivity as we turn to screens—forsaking (among other things) quiet rest, simple artistry, artful husbandry, and sustained concentration. We buy into what Wendell Berry calls the doctrine of general human limitlessness: although there is no such thing as a limitless animal, we believe humans are the exception. Berry warns that this thinking leads us to grasp for limitless possessions, knowledge, science, technology, and progress, which can only lead to limitless violence, waste, war, and destruction.

A woefully skewed picture of the world emerges, in which limited humans can literally make all life on the planet disappear, including our own. Clinging to vain delusions of limitlessness, we hasten our ultimate limit: death. Whether it is the harm done to our bodies through disrupted sleep or the breathtaking extermination of entire ecosystems, when we assume a boundlessness that is never ours to attain, we court disintegration. Perhaps Father James did know something about the way the world worked, after all. When we forsake darkness, when we try to do away with the night (or any earthbound equilibrium, for that matter), we are seeking to be something we are not—that illusive limitless animal.

I moved from pondering Father James's wisdom to revisiting the Apostle Paul's famous Love Hymn, in which he offers a magnificently obscure image of seeing in a "mirror dimly" or, in the King James, "glass darkly": "For now we see in a mirror, dimly, but then we will see face to face. Now I know only in part; then I will know fully, even as I have been fully known." Rather than a spiritual liability, the dark glass invites seers to spiritual maturity, to put away childish visions of the world and its gods as simple and knowable—whose thoughts mirror one's own. The dark glass engenders humility. Since we don't know it all, we need others. Seasoned believers do not bemoan the dim mirror, because they understand that obscurity is necessary to growth.

In Christian mystical traditions, darkness is integral to the soul's journey—a positive spiritual good, not a malevolent force to be eradicated or exorcised. Darkness prepares believers for divine encounter. St. John of the Cross, a sixteenth-century Spanish mystic, details the journey that readies the soul to receive God. On the path toward divine union, one must undergo a period of purgation and preparation—the "dark night of the soul"—wherein the soul is "made ready for the inestimable delights of the love of God." While the dark night is profoundly stripping and painful as the soul is "purified in this furnace like gold in a crucible," the darkness is not evil. To the contrary, John calls it "this happy night," which marks an "inflowing of God into the soul." The dark night, this *happy* night, is a necessary passage on the way to complete receptivity of the divine.

Darkness, however, is no mere stopover on the way to a more dazzling estate; darkness is one's dwelling place. "The darkness is enough," writes the Trappist monk Thomas Merton. It is the last line of a prayer he penned in the black hours before Midnight Mass on Christmas 1941, two weeks after he had entered the Abbey at Gesthemani. Darkness is not only sufficient, it is also liberating. "The night, O my Lord, is a time of freedom," Merton notes, reflecting upon his nighttime rounds as the fire watcher for the monastery. "[T]he night was never made to hide sin, but only to open infinite distances to charity and send our souls to play beyond the stars." Such endorsements of the night disrupt flimsy spiritual formulations that equate darkness with ignorance or evil.

•

In 2010, four years before my grandfather's death, I had a transformative experience with darkness, and its complementary relationship to light, atop Mount Sinai. I admit, a minister claiming to have had a religious encounter on Mount Sinai is a bit "on the nose." My story, however, is not supernatural; my face did not shine, nor did I receive tablets of divine commands. At the time, I did not have the words to describe what had so moved me, but as I reconsidered the metaphor of darkness in the months after Jack's funeral, my memories of Mount Sinai took on a new clarity.

Our ascent of the mountain began at 1:00 a.m., with a faint tapping at the door. Ryan and I, and our friends Matt and Hana, were sound asleep after a long day on a hot bus, winding through the streets of metropolitan Cairo, slowly passing through the Suez checkpoint, bribing our way through military outposts in the Sinai Peninsula, and finally settling in at St. Catherine's Monastery at the base of Mount Sinai. The knocking persisted, grew louder.

"Matt, is that the guide?" Ryan asked.

"It's too early," Matt groused. He rolled out of bed, cracked the door, muttered some Arabic, closed the door.

"He wants to leave now," Matt announced.

Yousef, our teenage Bedouin guide, had come to fetch us much earlier than we had planned. He said it would be better if we did not wait until later. He did not say why taking off at such an ungodly hour was preferable. It just was, and it seemed wise for us to trust him. From our sleep, we quickly arose and began our nighttime ascent of the mountain—in the pitch black, in the cold, with only the slobbery snorts and shit-smell of camels and the dim light of Yousef's iPod keeping us on the narrow path. Yousef glided effortlessly in sandals upon the rocky earth.

Muffling our heavy breathing and ignoring the sweat that turned to icy scales on our foreheads and chins, we made no complaint as we trailed Yousef's faint light and passed other pilgrims (many on camelback) as if they were standing still. The next day, we met a young American tourist, who said that it had taken him a full three hours to scale the mountain. Yousef had us to the top in half that time.

The last leg of the journey involved following tiny lights, held by old Bedouin men, who crouched near the ground, illumining steep, narrow stone steps—courtesy or perhaps emergency lighting for those who had made it this far. Yousef pointed to the rocky, vertical path, "go here," then he and his light disappeared. His vanishing, which he executed so nonchalantly, unsettled me; when one travels an alien path, the absence of a guide can feel like an eternity. Once we had made it to the top—at this point, there was no masking our heavy breathing—Yousef reappeared, looked at us with what I read as judgment—*what took you so long?*—and led us to a small stone wall at the edge of the mountain. He motioned for us to sit right along the ledge, and disappeared again. A small group of Bedouins camped nearby, but otherwise we were alone on the ledge. We shivered, huddled together for warmth, and waited in darkness. I had never felt so awake.

Soon we understood why Yousef knocked on our door at 1:00 a.m. and why he had fast-tracked us up the mountain. As dawn approached, other pilgrims began arriving in droves; our once-private enclave by the stone wall soon became crowded. It was clear we had some of the best seats on the mountain—no one in front of us, nothing between us and the horizon. I was irritated by the late-coming German tourists who pressed in behind me. I turned my head back toward them to scowl: that was the last trifling moment I remember.

I turned back to the wilderness. The hour had come. A banquet of arid pleasures spread out before us: desert mountains and desert valleys and the sky's refractive arc. A swelling luminosity touched thick darkness, unveiling the barren grandeur of peaks and plains. Ridges converted from dark slate to deep indigo to creamy crimson; the lowlands followed in kind. Night and day held each other, a slow embrace of blues and golds: hues of grace—gilded light finding home, complement, and balance in cerulean darkness. The two met in the thinnest of margins, at the slivered brink of bald horizon. Honored equals paying homage to their common source, each passed through the other—awakening me from, as Merton put it, "a dream of separateness." In a twinkling of an eye, the binding of light and dark in universal substance released me from estrangement from the earth, from myself—held me in a beauty and truth that won't go into words. And just as quickly as it came, it was gone—the union hidden again, light in clear ascendency. Dark and light, out of their fusion, delivered the other back to distinction: a circadian movement so endogenous to the earth's body, so mystifying to my own. "We need to return to being two," writes the poet Mahmoud Darwish, "so we can go on embracing each other."

We soon stopped shuddering and shed our jackets as the sun overtook the mountaintop. Now the risen sun shone brighter than I had ever seen at six in the morning, as bright as any noonday sun. I squinted as I made my way down to the valley—now able to see the narrow mountain passes, the hair-pin twists and turns, from which the dark night had mercifully shielded me. For a few privileged moments, atop Sinai, I stood in that place between night and the edge of light—endured a peace approaching perfect, desiring neither defeat for the dark nor triumph for the light. The moment of contact was enough. The two becoming one, then parting again, only to prepare for another reunion.

Mount Sinai was not the first place I had encountered that thin place between light and dark. At the other end of the world, at the other end of the day, I had become familiar with this edge. In reverse negative to night on the edge of dawn, this edge was between daylight and the edge of darkness. Here, too, equanimity emerges. The sub-suburban neighborhood of my childhood was the site of my initiation into what I came to know as the "golden hour."

I grew up in a split-level house, in a neighborhood erected in the 1970s, in a 10,000-person town outside the 35,000-person Cape Girardeau. The subdivision used to be a family farm. After developers bulldozed the old farmhouse (that we kids thought was haunted and ugly simply because it was not new), the only remnants of the farm were the street signs, which bore the names of members of the farm family. We lived on the patriarch's Otto Drive. Our backyard bumped up against his daughter's Charlotte Court, which intersected with his wife's Donna Drive. Otto neighbors surrounded us to the sides and front, Charlotte neighbors hemmed us in from behind, and we sat in easy view of houses on Donna. We possessed only enough privacy to qualify as true suburbia.

In our squeezed backyard, my dad constructed a camouflage tent, just tall enough for him to stand in and just wide enough to fit his tripod. The tent consisted of a skeleton of interlocking PVC pipes covered by an army tarp. It had a slit to walk through and a cutout window flap the size of a sheet of notebook paper. I rarely entered the tent; my dad made clear that it was no playhouse for kids. A permanent fixture in our yard, it sat entirely out of place among the usual Otto-Charlotte-Donna yard ornaments: bird baths, pansy planters, the occasional resin Virgin. The neighbors knew about my dad's hobby, which did not alleviate my embarrassment. Why couldn't he be like other subdivision dads, who worked outside only in the interest of lawn maintenance and house repairs? After dinner, he retreated to his tent to take photographs of birds—and also, no doubt, to decompress from his daily work in law enforcement. He extended the telephoto lens through the window flap and waited in solitude.

For a time, I thought his evening photo sessions were out of utility; since he worked during the day, after dinner was the only pocket of time he had to shoot. But not entirely so. One day he told me about the golden hour—the small period of morning and evening light that makes for the best photos. Because the early morning's golden hour—the one I would later experience on Mount Sinai—was lost to work and school schedules (and my dad was never a morning person), I came to know the golden hour as primarily an evening occurrence. Whereas daylight shines too directly to capture subtlety, the golden hour, also known as the "magic hour," warms a subject and renders it in proper texture, unleashing its full splendor. Direct sun sharpens the contrast between light and dark, creating deep pockets of shadow amid unforgiving brightness. Midday light can become so penetrative that it can lap itself: harsh contrasts give way to no contrast; the light scorches a subject, burning away its contours, which lends a washed-out quality to the image. Golden hour glow, conversely, releases subjects from harsh disparities, softening the shadows without being rid of them, holding the subject in tender embrace. Whereas midday sun beats down, golden hour light comes at a slant. More horizontal than vertical, it is egalitarian light. The light/dark dualism, so stark in the high beam of midday, recedes in the golden hour. Illumination and shadow converge, working in tandem to create a complex yet singular image.

My dad's birds hung, framed, on our walls: luminous goldfinches, hummingbirds and their intricately hued wings, the auburn breasts of blue birds—all tendered in warm and won-drous relief, courtesy of the golden hour and my dad's patient eye. While the rest of the neighbors stayed indoors, faces lit up by flickering screens that droned the same apocalyptic news, my father nested in his self-made tent I had thought so embarrassing—waiting in quiet dusk to capture the delicacies of flight and nuptial plumage in transfiguring light.

"The golden hour." Somehow that phrase also leads me back to the summer after my college freshman year, the last summer of the millennium. A charismatic professor had convinced me to study abroad, despite my reservations. I would be the first person in my immediate family to go abroad; it would be my first time flying alone, which frightened me; and I wondered if the course, "Victorian London," was worth it.

One evening, I walked the hills of London's Hampstead Heath searching for John Keats's house. I was nineteen and of late had discovered Keats—his aching heart, his pen drip-ping with beauty and truth, and his specter-thin tubercular death at twenty-five. In the falling light, I came to what may have been his home; I remember little of the structure, only the ending of day, old streets and old trees, and a peppering of despair. A small-town Midwestern girl, four thousand miles across land and sea from Otto Drive, searching for Keats in London's soft-dying day, I was shot through with sorrowful comprehension, noting in my journal: *By Keats's timeline, I have six more years to live, love, write. He dwelled with a beauty that must die, and so do I, so must I.* All my life—even at nineteen—I had been prone to pregnant moments like these, what I now describe as "golden hour" moments, when the thin edge between life and death presses upon me, waking me from a drowsy numbness. There are times in a day and a life—moments that can only be witnessed, never willed—when the inimitable heart of the universe swells across gulfs that seem impassable in ordinary time.

Tender is the night—that small, arresting phrase in Keats's "Ode to a Nightingale"—has made a new kind of sense to me as I've revisited my golden hour experiences. Defying dominant currents that equate black with deviance and darkness with violence, Keats offers the night that heartbreaking word: "tender." Sensitive, soft, gentle. The cutting, contrastive noonday light gives way to the tender night. The tender night brings peace. It rounds sharp edges, blunting the blade that slices up the world, hastily dividing wheat from chaff, worthy from unworthy. The night invites surrender, a release of control, as we cease separating the world for a time. Keats's night, that "embalmed darkness" in which he hears the lone nightingale's song, calls him to a middling place between wakefulness and sleep, where he is "half in love with easeful Death." Sleeping and waking find tender embrace. Death and life are loved in equal measure; neither is resisted. The golden hour provides passage to and from this tender night.

———

Might golden hours offer a much-needed antidote to the idea of golden years? Golden years make for disappointment. I have heard many times, through tears and gritted teeth, at the bedside, at the graveside: "These were *supposed* to be the golden years." But instead illness, chronic pain, financial woes, family strife, dementia, death, life's usual contradictions, have cut them short or taken them away. And golden years—the idea of them—so often function, I think, as future reward, as the prize for staying dutiful and harried in the decades preceding them. Golden hours, however, might draw us more deeply *into*, instead of *away from*, the present moment. By no effort of our own do we bring about golden hours. Rather, we receive them, allowing them to touch us, to move us to greater knowing. Awakening us to impermanence, they come and go whether or not anyone takes note of their fleeting beauty. Golden hours help us to see ourselves, others, and our surroundings by a certain generous luminosity balanced by darkness.

I recall a son who sat with his mother in an alcove bathed in natural light at the end of the dementia unit hallway. He would slowly flip a photo album, balancing it between them. Sometimes he pointed to a picture and offered a word of commentary, but mostly he was quiet. His mother looked content. Almost every afternoon they sat together in this manner. The son said of their practice: "If you wait long enough, something always comes." I was the new chaplain to the place at that time, new to the immense grace found in these moments of encounter. I have since taken his wisdom as a kind of initiation, a baptism into my work with persons who have dementia. *If you wait long enough, something always comes.* You must wait, long, enough. I tried to understand this waiting in the manner in which Thoreau understood certain still days he spent in the woods, as "not time subtracted from your life, but so much over and above your usual allowance."

•

My grandfather had enjoyed center stage, relished the spotlight. Whether he was singing solos in church, or serving as the Rotarian state governor, or organizing a veterans group and writing its newsletters, Jack was unafraid of prominence. Always working on important projects, always instructing, always on the move, his transparent passion made him radiant.

I admired my grandfather but did not feel close to him. He seemed always above, remote—on stage. By design, stage lighting makes it easy for the audience to see the actors and hard for the actors to see the audience. I felt like the approving audience member, always seeing but never really being seen, and he—the faraway performer—was always being seen but never really seeing beyond the stage. My grandmother once told me that she saw her role as the "hand-clapper" for her husband; she said this as a point of fact, not contention. She likely felt the spectator's distance, too.

Not long after we were married in 2002, Ryan and I visited my grandparents. My grandfather played one of his Three Tenors albums on his stereo at the highest volume imaginable, nearly blasting us out of the room. (Although his hearing was bad, it was not *that* bad.) He stood and sang along operatically, making sweeping hand motions and lifting his head high—as if he were the fourth tenor. He took out his trombone from its case and played a few measures for us, as we sat on the ottoman, knees close to chest, staring up at him like schoolchildren. Although there were certain oddities to the visit that probably pointed to early signs of dementia—he had some trouble working his stereo and finding certain words—the performance, the show-and-tell aspects of the visit, were not so unusual, if somewhat amplified. What *was* new: for the first time I felt the weight of the stage's obstructive distance, the strain it placed on our adult relationship. I sat, still and heavy as a millstone, politely applauding Jack next to my clapping husband—aware of an enduring gap that may never close.

Years later, in my grandfather's late dementia, I experienced a new tenderness in him, as the spotlights darkened and the houselights softly came up. He was no longer on stage. He was in a wheelchair. He lived in a nursing home where no one knew him from any other old veteran. He did not speak much. He hummed on occasion. My memories of him in these months are candlelit: the circle of light he emanated was small but warm. A new stillness eclipsed his earlier frenetic disposition. At first, it was hard to receive this new faintness as a gift; it was hard for my eyes to adjust to darkening after staring into such brightness for so long. It was hard to see anything at all. But once I adjusted to the lower light, I felt a kind of exhalation: relief. For the first time in my life, I sat with my grandfather, eye to eye, no showing, no telling, no clapping. While his past light had beamed, attracting my attention and admiration but rarely my affection, his new darkling light was inviting, even gentle.

I've wondered if one reason Jack appears so frequently in my writing is my effort to unpack the surprising trajectory of our relationship. Aren't I supposed to tell of my growing sense of alienation from my once-close loved one, whose dementia now drives a wedge between us? However, our last visits together are more memorable and engaging to me, tug more at my inner cords, than any other time I spent with him. The distance between us felt, for once and at last, bridgeable—as his lighting no longer crowded out his subtler shades and no longer crowded out me. I could finally see him as through a glass dimly, not blinded by the bright glare. And maybe he could see me beside him, not as an entranced audience member but as a friend in the waning light. In those final months, light seemed to find parity in dark. No longer a spellbound spectator, perhaps I was on the stage, too—a kind of stagehand, like Houdini's assistant Dorothy, attending to the motions of another's vanishing.

On the afternoon of my last visit with my grandfather before his death, we sat outside together—he in his wheelchair, me on a bench—watching that pin oak in the front lawn of the Veterans Home. All of my attempts to converse with him failed, and this silence that had originally made me squirm drove me to simply sit for a while and try to listen. Flags waved along the driveway, cars passed in the distance, and birds flitted between branches. The shadows grew longer and longer, nightfall's hour grew nearer and nearer, but seemed not to reach us yet. My initial discomfort with the stillness gave way to a passing peace. The soft sounds, the stretches of silence, the coming of the golden hour, soothed the sting of coming departures.

From the grounds of his rural Kentucky monastery, Merton writes of communion with the divine as being "[e]ngulfed in the simple and lucid actuality of the afternoon—I mean God's afternoon." It is in the sinking light—what he calls "this sacramental moment of time when the shadows will get longer and longer"—in which he feels a special confirmation of his call to solitude. After noting the simple and lucid actualities—"one small bird sings quietly in the cedars, one car goes by in the remote distance, and the oak leaves move in the wind [. . .]"— Merton declares, "The more I am in it, the more I love it. One day it will possess me entirely and no man will ever see me again." The elongating shadows of the afternoon confirm Merton's calling; the day's darkening delivers him to solitude. Merton exults in sylvan holiness. Birdsong, cedars, wind, leaves, a lone car—the simple constituents of what he calls a day that "goes by in prayer." Merton desires the growing shade to overtake him, to possess him so entirely that he merges with it, vanishes into it—until "no man will ever see me gain." No longer a distinct, separate entity, Merton imagines a complete merger into the sacrament of the moment, the afternoon solitude, *God*.

The next time I saw Jack, he was in peaceful repose, in a gray suit in his coffin, stiller than still, possessed entirely, never to be seen again.

•

I am seeing again my visit to the sculpture park in central New Jersey. By the time I had stepped out of Seward Johnson's rendering of *The Dream*, the evening had grown late, reaching the tail end of the golden hour. It was too dark for photos without the stark intrusion of a flash. It was just light enough to see tracings of the landscape but not its thousands of departures that make *this* not *that*. The points of separation receded with the falling light as the darkening world ascended into palpable unity. The aboveground roots appeared as small dark waves. The tree branches bent, one touched the other and another. It was hard to track which limbs swayed where, when; I mostly knew by wind sound, less and less by sight. The tips of the branches, their small leaves, converged into singular silhouette, in concert with itself.

On my way to the park's exit, I rounded the bend to discover

Seward Johnson's interpretation of Matisse's *The Dance*: swirling women in an interlocking circle, each curvy nude reflecting and holding the other—a world without end. Each bare woman stood eight feet tall, cast in aluminum; together, they formed a towering union, an especially large ring. Johnson gave the title *Daydream* to his spin on *The Dance*. In his rendition, he has added a reclining man in the middle of the circle, arms behind his head, staring lustily up at the dancing women.

I stepped over the lying daydreamer and stood beneath the whirl, wide-eyed under their soaring embrace. The lengthening shadow of their yoked arms enclosed me, as we slow danced the light away, making way for the happy night.

6

A Great Many
Seemings Here

HERE IS A PARTIAL LIST OF THINGS I'VE DONE IN MY sleep: I have pushed my heavy chest of drawers along the bedroom wall because it was blocking the doorway and my parents were trying to get in. I have stripped my bed of its top blanket because houseguests who were sleeping in the living room needed it. I have taken a shower at two in the morning because it was time to go to work. I have frantically searched the apartment for my friend's baby because I had forgotten to care for her. I have slept on the couch because a snake was in my bed. I have cleaned the bathroom counter because visitors were arriving. I have unpacked the first aid kit because a house-guest had cut herself. Of course, there were no actual parents, houseguests, babies, snakes, or visitors. The chest did not block the doorway; it was not time for work; no one was forgotten or injured.

Ryan has tried to ask me, while I am sleepwalking, what I am doing and why, but I am never able to explain my reality in any kind of traditional narrative. Instead, I use indistinct language: "I'm just trying to get it," "They're coming soon," or "Is it gone yet?" Because I mostly use pronouns (it, she, they), Ryan has to guess to what reality they point. When I am sleep-walking, I live by impressions, of this or that *seeming* this or that way—rather than by well-defined story lines. A vague dream scenario elicits a palpable feeling and compels me to act. I have reasons for acting, but I am foggy on the details. The particu-lars remain obscure. I have an impression, not a precise picture. For instance, with the first aid kit incident, I possessed a strong notion that someone was hurt in my apartment and I needed to help. I did not have a clear sense why the visitor—a female friend of mine, it seemed—was bleeding, nor did I see or inter-act with her. My dream logic went something like this: *There seems to be someone in our apartment. Someone I seem to know. Someone who seems to need something. Oh, yes, it seems my friend is here. And, oh no, it seems she is hurt . . . cut . . . bleeding! I should do something. Yes, the first aid kit in the linen closet. I will place it somewhere . . . where can she see it? The kitchen table. There does not seem to be anything else I should do. It seems I should go back to bed.*

Ryan used to try to correct me in my sleep states: "There's nothing there," "Come back to bed," "Don't do that." These interventions rarely worked. His attempts at orienting me left me feeling hurt or embarrassed, and I still felt compelled to respond to my dreamworld reality. Ryan has learned I respond better to validation: "Everything is taken care of," or "I'll get it in the morning." Mostly, however, he has learned not to interfere while I am having an episode. I have never hurt myself or anyone else, and I typically return to bed within a few minutes. If Ryan remains a detached observer, often he can collect funny stories to tell later—like when I declared, with lawyer-like authority, as I stood in our bedroom doorway: "I have never tried cocaine, so we can rule that out!" Or, when I sat up in bed and said, "These are so big. Can I hold them?" The latter is among his favorite episodes to recount, for obvious and juvenile reasons.

I once stayed the night with a friend who became so upset when she found out that I was a sleepwalker that she was afraid to go to sleep, afraid I would do something to her. She thought I would mutate into something ghastly. Non-sleepwalkers often harbor such fears. I seldom sleepwalk in the presence of anyone other than Ryan or in places outside my own home. Like most sleepwalkers, my sense of place and time is fuzzy, if not wholly amiss, yet my sense of self remains intact. I do not lose inhibition; I do not act radically out of character. I possess motives, even if strange or convoluted. I am more remote, seeming far off or fragmented, than I am reckless or startling or even irrational. Later, I often can remember some details of my sleepwalking episodes, especially if Ryan prompts me the next morning with something I said or did. I am in a middling space: I am neither fully awake (or I would abandon my course of action), nor am I fully asleep (or I would recall little to nothing the next morning). While I can access some of my feelings and motives, some bits and pieces from my walking dream, I am not able to weave them together into a singular and stable account. The episode remains slippery in my memory. The narrative refuses solidity.

Curiously enough, sleepwalking gave me new eyes for Claude Monet. On museum trips, I used to either skip the Monet paintings altogether or make only a brief pass by them. Monet had struck me as too pastoral, too soft and lovely, to offer the gut reaction for which I longed. I gravitated instead to the Fauves like Matisse and the Abstract Expressionists like Rothko and de Kooning, who seemed bolder and more immediate. I associated Monet's work with the pastel patterns on Kleenex boxes, and Impressionism with the presumably safe and pretty art style I learned, to the exclusion of others, in secondary school.

On a recent trip to New York's Museum of Modern Art, during a perfunctory pass by Monet's huge three-panel *Water Lilies*, I had a gut reaction. It was substantial. The painting flowed, and I flowed within it. I knew the water lilies like I knew my dreams: not by strict realism, but by their movement within a larger field. *Water Lilies* impressed me, not by its precision but by its plasticity. The play of light, splashes of color, patterns of strokes corresponded to the fluid associations, the loose yet connected composition, of my sleepwalking episodes. "In the attempt to capture the constantly changing qualities of natural light and color," read the museum's description, "spatial cues all but dissolve; above and below, near and far, water and sky all commingle." The aim of his *Water Lilies* triptych, Monet said, was to give "the illusion of an endless whole, of water without horizon or bank." While spatial cues all but dissolve in *Water Lilies*, the result is not unreason or chaos but an intricate, expansive unity. Similarly, as traditional narrative cues all but dissolve in my sleepwalking, the result is not unreason or chaos. Each of my dreaming notions is like a Monet lily— floating, fluid, yet part of a larger whole. I follow inner motions, blurry yet strangely related. Emotion and compulsion, desire and action, the conscious and unconscious, all commingle. In Monet's world, I saw my sleepwalking self exquisitely reflected back to me. Like water without horizon or bank, the ephemerality of my dreams defies apparent boundaries.

The more I worked with people with dementia at the Gardens and spent time with my grandfather, the more I longed to connect with their experiences—to move beyond simple projection or pity, and find some way to feel within myself a bit of what they might feel. While I do not presume I can or should know in full the experiences of another, I wondered if sleepwalking might be one point of correspondence. Accounts written by people with dementia seem to suggest some similarity. "With my memory systems as they are, simple recollection is as fluid as waking from a dream, with things that I believe to be vital vanishing as I reach for them," writes the essayist Floyd Skloot, who suffered brain damage at forty-one from a viral infection. In his memoir, *In the Shadow of Memory*, Skloot describes the feeling of forgetting as "still eerie," although it has become normal to him. Skloot says he knows intimately what the Harvard professor of psychiatry J. Allan Hobson means when he writes, "the poor memory we have of dreams once we awaken from them is similar to the memory lapses experienced by Alzheimer's patients." Like Skloot, Christine Bryden compares the slipperiness of her own dementia to the ambiguity experienced in semi-sleep states—further corroborating Hobson's description of memory loss. In her autobiography, *Dancing with Dementia: My Story of Living Positively with Dementia*, Bryden describes herself as "caught between dreams and daily life," inhabiting a world "between sleep and awake," filled with "dark shapes" and "real feelings." Within this dissolving and commingling, she often finds herself wondering, "So what is real, what is true?"

Aspects of dementia experiences—at least for some people—resemble dream states. This correlation, perhaps, comes as little surprise, since both conditions involve altered perception. Nevertheless, it carries profound implications. For those of us who do not have dementia yet, our experiences of dreaming could serve as rare empathic portals to the world of dementia. Sleepwalking could, perhaps, help me understand what others feel like—what *I* might feel like when I have dementia. Sleepwalking opens me to a domain ruled more by emotional impressions, by a world of dark shapes and real feelings and its own hazy logic, than by the dictates of apparent reason. Meaning does not evaporate, even as traditional narratives do. When walking in a sleep state I may grow shifted, fragmented, foggy, but I do not cease feeling or desiring or even thinking—and, if the comparison holds, neither do persons with dementia.

While at times sleepwalking can be distressing to me, depending upon the nature of my dream, it is not *always* so—and certainly not always acutely so. The response to my sleepwalking can often ameliorate or exacerbate my distress. How Ryan reacts to me deeply influences how I feel about my inner experience. This dialectic gives me a small glimpse into the day-to-day plight of someone living with dementia: how her social world's response to her affects whether she feels embarrassed or affirmed, dismissed or heard, human or inhuman.

In addition to the surface similarities between dementia and dreaming, the rhetorical correlation of dreaming and dementia holds promise, too. Descriptions of dementia that draw upon dream analogies seem to move away from the horror-tinged depictions of people with dementia as losing their minds or vacating their bodies, as enduring "death in slow motion" or an "endless funeral." Dreaming does not necessarily inspire dread; rather, dreaming is considered a part of life, albeit one of its stranger manifestations. Dreamers do not endure social stigma, humiliation, or ostracization. To the contrary, dreaming metaphors often invoke tender, even spiritual, qualities.

Dream language infuses descriptions of Ralph Waldo Emerson, who lived the final decade of his life with progressive forgetfulness. Julian Hawthorne, the novelist Nathaniel Hawthorne's son, writes of Emerson, a longtime family friend and neighbor, during the final year of Emerson's life: "His face, in these times was quiescent, as one who dreams awake." Speaking with Emerson, Julian writes, "was like conversing through a veil." Emerson reminds him of "an angel half asleep." Julian calls Emerson's state a "semi-spiritual retreat." "The light of the passing day was as a mirage to him," he writes. Charles Norton, another friend of Emerson, notes, "[A]t times his mind moves as in dreams."

These dream-inflected descriptors paint Emerson's disposition as vague yet serene. He exists in a mystical dream—not an unrelenting nightmare. His new vulnerability strikes Julian as "touching" and "in no respect a painful spectacle." The journalist William Dean Howells, after seeing a forgetful Emerson give a lecture, comments that he was beginning "to achieve an identity independent of memory" and that this was a "gift of purely spiritual continuity." By these accounts, the afflicted Emerson remains spiritually vital and fully human—as one who, simply and even quite divinely, "dreams awake."

Just as the literal points of comparison between dreaming

and dementia have limits—dreamers have the distinct privilege of waking up; sleepwalking is neither progressive nor terminal—rhetorical comparisons have their limits, too. Dreaming—like all dementia metaphors—carries its own potentially harmful baggage. If we imagine that those with dementia live in a sleepy dreamworld, then those without dementia must live in the awakened *real* world. The correlation between dreaming and dementia could reinforce a crude divide between dreaming/demented and awake/nondemented. By this logic, people with dementia are not candidates for sustained and sincere engagement any more than wandering sleepers are. After all, they (and they alone) live in and by illusions. We can humor them and help them, but we need never treat them as fully human or credible.

In his writings, Emerson—that waking dreamer himself—offers a powerful corrective for this asymmetry. "Dream delivers us to dream, and there is no end to illusion," he writes in his 1844 essay "Experience." Thirteen years later, in "Illusions," he puts it this way: "We wake from one dream into another dream." A treatise on changeability, "Illusions" asserts that life is riddle and illusion all the way down, for all of us. There are no finalities; rather, all is "loose and floating" and subject to "incessant flowing and ascension." The anchors of perception prove impermanent. We live in a perpetual state of unknowing, moving from dream to dream, in which "the capital facts of human life are hidden from our eyes." Try as we might, "[w]e cannot write the order of the variable winds."

The Emersonian vision places us all in the world of illusions, thereby softening the harsh divide between "real" and "dream" worlds. Illusions cover universal human ground, and this common cover could help us to reimagine dementia. If we accept our own perceptions, now, as dream upon dream, we can locate dementia experiences along the continuum of human experience, rather than as alien or aberrant behavior. We can no longer consign them (the dreamers, the "demented") to unreality, any more than we can lay exclusive claim to reality. We, both people who have dementia and people who do not have dementia yet, traffic in layers of illusions.

Perhaps the cognitive fragmentation of people with dementia simply renders visible the illusory nature of all knowing. The slipperiness of their perceptions often emerges in overt, recognizable ways. A friend's name is forgotten; a pineapple is called a pear; the time of year is unknown. As usual modes of communication increasingly elude them, their "baffled intellects"—a curiously fitting Emerson phrase—are laid bare, exposing the loose and floating quality of the mind. Because our illusions remain more discrete and conform to social norms—and do not originate from "brain damage"—those of us without dementia more easily hold the illusion that we do not live by illusions. Whereas our partial and skewed perceptions may grind on—unshaken and affirmed by our social worlds for decades—their misperceptions immediately and directly confound their interactions with others. While I may not forget the word for pear or confuse my husband for my brother, I may

believe other, more damaging and ubiquitous illusions, such as
I am safe; tomorrow will resemble today; you get what you deserve.

·

At the beginning of "Illusions," Emerson reflects upon his 1850
trip to Mammoth Cave. At the end of the tour, Emerson and
his fellow travelers have their lights taken from them and ex-
tinguished. Overhead, on the cave's ceiling, it seems as if stars
twinkle against the dark of outer space. The party is astonished
and delighted. Emerson soon discovers the spectacle's source:
a half-hid lamp; its light, refracted by crystal formations embedded in the cave, creates the cosmic illusion. Our sensory
perceptions, Emerson asserts, always interfere with our experiences: "Our conversation with Nature is not just what it
seems." *Seems*: gives the impression, appears, looks *as if.* The
word is load-bearing: living by illusions means we live by seeming, by shifting moods, by ebbing and flowing impressions.

Two days before Christmas 2015, on a cross-country trip
from the East Coast to Missouri, I took a detour, dipping into
southern Kentucky to visit Mammoth Cave National Park.
One hundred and sixty-five years after Emerson's trip, I entered Mammoth, too, but I had no need to bring my own light.
Lightbulbs enclosed by wire fixtures dotted the cave walls, cast-
ing a soft glow on the formations. Calcite deposits rusted the
landscape; coppery striations coated the walls, lining them like
an ulcerated stomach. Backlit stalagmites and stalactites—that

pair perennially confused on fourth-grade science quizzes—created watery shadows. I saw the formations, much as a fourth grader might, as large towers of mashed potatoes. Our guide pointed to rock clusters on the wall: the long, thin "soda straws" and the small, knotty "popcorn." He spotlighted the green algae growing next to the popcorn. It does not grow here naturally, he explained. Humans brought in spores on the soles of their shoes, and the algae grew by the heat of the incandescent lights. The newly installed LED lightbulbs promise to inhibit the patches' growth.

The guide moved his beam to leggy, slow-moving cave crickets whose bodies appeared transparent, wholly colorless, against the dark layer of their own dung beneath them. He showed us tubular indentations in the limestone, a network of seams that looked like small tree roots, each tract barely finger-width. "Each seam will one day be a new chamber, as large as the one we are standing in," the guide declared, as if this were not earth-shattering news. I wondered what would become of the chamber in which we then stood.

Mammoth is the largest known cave system in the world. As of this writing, four hundred miles of continuous cave, a network of hallowed spaces, stacked and winding, have been discovered. Our guide likened the labyrinthine Mammoth to an upside-down plate of spaghetti. Possessing no lexicon for the cave's weirdness, we curiously resort to banal comparisons with starchy foods. Perhaps such food-based analogies attach themselves only naturally to this great stone belly.

Swallowed up by the earth's *crust*, we find ourselves in its dark and ghostly gut.

We arrived in a rare part of the cave where groundwater penetrates the sandstone shelf above the cave's limestone and cascades through an opening in the ceiling. Underground, I was splashed by a waterfall, descending through and from the ground I had just stood upon. I understood why Emerson began his discussion of illusions in a cave: questions of perception pressed in on me. Remnants of an old ocean, Mammoth is all still flowing; in geologic time, it swells and shifts, turning and returning to canyons, riverbeds, plains, sea floors. At once, I was walking upon the sunken floor of a drained ocean, descending the grim craters of Pluto, arriving in the shadowy depths of Sheol to congregate with the desireless dead. As if my eyes had been turned upside down, the world appeared flipped, heading at once forward and backward, up and down: Paleozoic and Anthropocene, the soles of rubber boots laced with algae spores, the rush of ancient rivers, the rise of continents, the handrails screwed to cave walls for balance. Was this great belly preparing to belch us out or to drive us deeper into the snaking intestines?

At the tour's end, before we made our ascent to the cave's entrance, our guide instructed us to close our eyes and to open them on his count. "*One.* Close your eyes," he instructed. "*Two.* I'm flipping off the lights. *Three.* Open your eyes." For a few seconds I observed the cave *as cave*, glimpsed the lightless majesty of inner space, before human intervention. Mammoth had been pitch black for millennia, its peculiar innards unseen—an endless whole, without horizon or bank. The group was quickly restless; a young child whimpered, "I'm scared." (At what point is what you see scarier than what you do not?) I wanted to stay in the dark for a long time—unseen and unseeing—but the lights soon returned, along with the outline of the cave's contents: ghastly crickets, murky forms, us. Was this the *real* and *true* Mammoth?

My Buddhist friend, who went to grade school in the '70s, said she always missed the questions on standardized tests that asked students to identify something as either an animal, vegetable, or mineral. She said she could always talk herself into and out of the categories, seeing elements of each in each. Does it not depend upon how far back one goes in the history of a particular formation's development, or how far forward one looks, or how interiorly? Is Mammoth an ocean, canyon, or cave?

At Christmas, my father—who loves nothing more than to impart a good piece of trivia—quizzed me on the largest living organism on the planet; I answered, "The crust of the earth?" He rolled his eyes, obviously disappointed: "I said *living!*" The correct answer was the blue whale, apparently. My husband disagreed, arguing for the honey fungus of Oregon's Blue Mountains. The riddle of perception confounds. The universe contains much more dark matter than luminous matter; the invisible outstrips the visible by six times. A grain of sand contains a whole world, I've heard. I've heard it's a matter of seeing.

——

When I was a hospital chaplaincy student, I learned to use the verb "seemed" when I made notes in patients' charts. I was not to write that the patient *was*, but that the patient *seemed*. The patient seemed angry, anxious, sad, fearful, peaceful, spiritually distressed, overwhelmed. The patient seemed to have an adequate (or inadequate) support system and resources for coping. The patient seemed to find meaning (or not) in religious practice. This noncommittal verb served as a buffer between the patient's experiences and my assessment of the patient's experiences. At the time, I didn't give much thought to its ubiquitous use. I assumed it reduced liability, since I was offering an informed impression—and not a diagnosis *per se*. But I've since come to appreciate how seemly seeming is, given that the power to apprehend is always partial, always yielding to riddle and illusion. Seeming is a gesture toward epistemological humility, toward the limits of what one can know. In the face of the incalculable human spirit, deference is indispensable. It seems it is best to keep seeming.

But we live in a world with little room for seeming. We want information. We want it fast. It must be immediately usable. Ten-word tweets count as culturally relevant contributions— and, of late, as a means for presidential pronouncements. We want the definitive. Acknowledging complexity and recommending prudence are anathema to the soundbite and the bullet point. The tedium of truth readily yields to the titillation of jingoism. We don't want things to *seem* this way or that—we want things to *be* all this way or all that: all good or all bad, all useful or all useless, all holy or all unholy. A person is sick or well, asleep or awake, confused or lucid. Seeming pushes back against such easy partitioning of the world.

Abiding uncertainty, Emerson maintains, need not spell moral apathy and its accompanying despair. Seeming does not discard the pursuit of truth or encourage intellectual laziness. Rather, it demands a sort of moral rigor. Just because we cannot write the order of the variable winds does not mean the universe is without order, for "all is system and gradation." We do not cease striving to penetrate illusions, to remove masks, to seek a more excellent way, however elusive, simply because we cannot lay hold of the ultimate or grasp the unfathomable. Illusions, according to Emerson, carry their own impetus toward the real, the true, the just: "If life seem a succession of dreams, yet poetic justice is done in dreams also." Never resting in present illusions, we aspire to loftier gradations of truth and justice.

Although we never achieve absolute clarity, Emerson holds out hope for moments when "the air clears, and the cloud lifts a little." In "Experience," he describes how these moments may provide glimpses of "a new and excellent region of life" in "flashes of light, in sudden discoveries of its profound beauty and repose." We do not dwell long in such intervals; we do not once and for all arrive, but rather we become apprised of "august magnificence." We approach this "vast-flowing vigor."

Always we are approaching. Even though human consciousness remains inconstant, there exists "that in us which changes not and which ranks all sensations and states of mind." "The baffled intellect," Emerson claims, bows before an "ineffable cause." This ineffable cause helps us to discern, discover, and generate profound beauty and repose—even as it resists categorization. An "unbounded substance," it "refuses to be named," he contends. Never a systematic thinker, Emerson himself refuses categorization, opting for opacity over a foolish consistency.

The "baffled intellect" became a terribly literal reality for Emerson in the last decade of his life when he experienced what Oliver Wendell Holmes, his earliest biographer, described as "the decline of his faculties." Emerson put it this way: "My memory hides itself." Emerson spoke of his memory loss as "vexation" and wished not to "afflict dear friends with my tied tongue." At other times, Emerson possessed humor about his deficits. When he could not remember the subject of a lecture he planned to give on education, he commented, "A funny occasion it will be—a lecturer who has no idea what he's lecturing about and an audience who don't know what he *can* mean!" In an 1880 correspondence with his friend Sam Bradford, Emerson wrote, "I rejoice to find you perfect in your memory, and master in your writing, while I have ceased to write, because the pen refuses to spell." True enough, he sent only three more brief letters.

His friends noted some of Emerson's clever circumlocutions when he could not recall certain words. Searching for the word "umbrella," he said, "I can't tell its name, but I can tell its history. Strangers take it away." He called railroads "those things that go to and fro" and a plow "the implement that cultivates the soil." Speaking of the nation's Capitol, he described it as "United States—survey of the beauty of eternal Government." "He penetrated beyond names," wrote William Henry Furness, referencing Emerson's aphasia, "and dealt only with realities." Despite his speech deficits, Emerson continued to give lectures, often with the help of his daughter Ellen. In 1881, the year before his death, he delivered his final public lecture. The scholar Joseph Slater describes the scene:

> He stumbled over long words. When he seemed
> entirely defeated, Ellen would make the sounds
> silently and he would imitate her lips. He read
> loudly enough for all to hear, but even so his
> audience drew closer into a circle around him.

His listening community, in a tender gesture of solidarity, hemmed him in.

One month before his death, in the depths of progressive forgetfulness, Emerson attended the funeral of his friend Henry Wadsworth Longfellow. After going to the casket twice, Emerson asked Ellen, "Where are we? What house? And who is the sleeper?" When she told him, he arose a third time and walked to the coffin to see Longfellow again. A fellow funeral-goer, Moncure Conway, reported that, upon seeing Longfellow, Emerson said, "That gentleman was a sweet, beautiful soul, but I have entirely forgotten his name."

Even as Emerson grew weaker in the final months of his life, he insisted on taking his usual evening walks. Reportedly, he took longer walks as he grew more restless, perhaps as words, spoken and written, became increasingly inaccessible to him. Eight days before his death, Emerson got caught in a rainstorm on one of these strolls, and soon after, an existing cold became pneumonia. In the first days of his illness, Emerson continued to get dressed and come downstairs and sit by the fireplace, even tending the fire and latching the windows in his usual way.

The pneumonia further compromised his fragile memory. On a couple of days, Emerson believed he was a visitor in someone else's home and felt compelled to make the journey home. In a letter to a family friend, Ellen wrote, "[A]gain and again we succeeded in convincing him that he was home which consoled him till he forgot it." On another occasion, Emerson worried about the family's finances. After her father tried at length to make himself understood, Ellen deciphered the word "bills," and she reassured him that the bills were paid and there was money in the bank and the house. Ellen reported that on one morning when her father "looked very sick" and was unsteady on his feet, a frustrated Emerson declared, "I hoped it would not come in this way. I would rather—fall—down cellar!" In another heartrending moment, Emerson uttered to his wife, Lidian, "Oh, that beautiful boy!"—presumably referring to their first son, Waldo, whose sudden death at age five had devastated Emerson. "I grieve that grief can teach me nothing," wrote Emerson two years after Waldo's death, revealing the soul-numbing depth of his loss—a loss that revisited him in his final days.

More typically, however, his dying days were shot through with affection and peace. When he could no longer come downstairs, he received visitors in his sickroom. Visits from his young grandchildren particularly delighted him. "The sight of the children [. . .] was sure to make Father smile," Ellen reported, "and he could say 'Good boy!' 'Good little girl!' always and sometimes a little more." Longtime friends paid him visits, too: "What Father said to them indicated that he regarded it as farewell [. . .] he tried to sum up the relation he had held with each through life, this was plain though he couldn't say two words of a sentence right." In his journals, Bronson Alcott recounted the bittersweet final visit with his companion: "[H]e took my hand affectionately and said in strong but broken accents: 'You have strong hold on life, and maintain it firmly' [. . .]"

In his final hours, gazing about the room from his bed, Emerson reportedly proclaimed that there were "a great many seemings here." His utterance feels at once cryptic and load-bearing. "This surface on which we stand," he writes in "Circles," "is not fixed but sliding." How palpable is this sliding, this seeming, in the transition from life to death. Circles overlap; this life and the next slide over the other in sacred intersection. Perhaps we dwell inside both circles at once; their crossing contains us. *A great many seemings here.* Smaller swirls and eddies spin into larger circulations. Seams widen, rushing outward to new and larger circles, to greater expanses of beauty and repose, and that without end.

Sometimes when I have visited people who are dying, their chambers have seemed full, teeming with terrific and transitory impressions. Boundaries of time and space seem to have dissolved for them, and rounds of passing visitors, seen only by the dying, seem to circulate. For someone as expansive and relational as Emerson, someone so committed to following his own genius and encouraging others to follow theirs, I can only imagine what a great cloud of witnesses accompanied him in the end. It seems only fitting that Emerson's friend Judge Hoar reported that Emerson's face at the time of his death "seemed to give a glimpse of the opening heavens." A great many seemings attended Emerson, inaugurating him into a greater circle, apprising him of newer and more excellent regions.

·

A longtime fan of Emerson's essays, I had not given much thought to his biography until I began writing this book, and recalled that he had what was probably Alzheimer's disease in his late life. I wondered what I might learn from looking closely at Emerson's final years, before the full-blown stigmatization of old age and memory loss in America. Emerson died in 1882, twenty-four years before Auguste Deter died in a mental institution from an infected bedsore. He died before senility became a diagnosable disease, before that disease became equated with the dread and horror we think of now.

With the rapid industrialization of late nineteenth-century America, what were once considered natural aspects of advanced age came to have pejorative meanings; the demands of the new marketplace stigmatized those who were not physically and mentally able to adequately participate in an increasingly complex and bureaucratized system. With the rise of the American middle class in the twentieth century, the behaviors and symptoms associated with dementia called into question, according to Jesse Ballenger, "the very personhood of those who exhibited them." The disease's stigma arose from the sufferers' inability "to carry off their role as a respectable middle class person," which entailed presenting a "stable and coherent self to others." Since respectability was defined by the norms of white society, and the assumption that rationality was the domain of white men, one's inability to carry off a middle-class role bore anxieties related to gender and race, too.

While Emerson's "decline of faculties" saddened him and his loved ones, I find little evidence that his affliction precipitated a fall from grace. The naturalist John Muir declared the late-life, aphasic Emerson "as serene as a sequoia, his head in the empyrean." Walt Whitman described his final visit with

Emerson, who spoke very little at this point, as "a long and blessed evening," finding his friend's "old clear-peering aspect quite the same." Barely having escaped the modern stigma attached to dementia and old age, Emerson appears to have had a relatively good life and death with dementia.

In his 2001 bestselling book *The Forgetting: Alzheimer's: Portrait of an Epidemic*, David Shenk writes about the late-life Emerson—at times, using vanishing metaphors like "waning crescent" and "vacant ghost" to describe him. In 2004, PBS made a documentary based on Shenk's book, and the online material that accompanied the film included this description of Emerson: "In the last years of his life, Ralph Waldo Emerson was so wracked by senility that the renowned author could not even pen his own name. Oddly, he seemed to accept the loss of what most would consider his greatest asset, his mind." While the portrait initially calls his acceptance "odd," it goes on to acknowledge that it really was not so odd, given Emerson's cultural milieu: "Emerson's acceptance of his memory loss probably had a lot to do with the thinking of the time. Until recently, people simply believed that elderly senility was a part of the aging process." These lines reveal perhaps more than they intend; they imply that Emerson was able to accept his memory loss in large part because it had not been medicalized yet. They subtly suggest that no such acceptance would be possible in our own time. Now we would diagnose Emerson and initiate him into dementia's special stigma. No longer a serene sequoia, Emerson would become another Alzheimer's victim, tragically "fading away." If only he had known what we know now—that he had a terrible disease—then surely this knowledge would have thwarted his acceptance of his condition. I wonder how, exactly, this is progress.

I worry there is little space for "seeming" when it comes to people with dementia; we define them by their defects and reduce them to disease stages. I regularly receive invitations to programs that target the caregivers of people at early, middle, or late stages of Alzheimer's—as if these stages solely or easily determine individual needs, remaining capacities, or emerging desires. The afflicted receive plans of care and drug regimens, participate in special programs, and move to special units. And while these strategies, in their noblest incarnations, aim to alleviate suffering, I fear that somewhere along the way we stop seeing people with dementia as variable and dynamic individuals and start seeing them as a homogenous group of "sufferers." We pass judgment on them as *diseased* and thus essentially *deficient*, leaving nothing to the unfolding or the unfathomable. I fear we stop seeing them as persons who *seem* and start seeing them as patients who *are*.

It is tempting to play up the tragic irony of Emerson's "decline of faculties" by contrasting his incoherence at his life's ending with his previous erudition. The reference to the "loss" of Emerson's "greatest asset, his mind" reveals this impulse. It is tempting to make the same obvious and sentimental rhetorical

move: the quintessential American scholar who cannot remember the word for umbrella, the champion of self-reliance
who requires his daughter's help to finish a lecture, the Sage
of Concord who does not know in whose house he dwells. He
makes a particularly pitiable victim, a fine example of dementia's ruthlessness: "If even *his* mind can go . . ." These descriptions are as dramatic as they are reductive. They are terribly
hard to resist. And yet I desperately want to resist.

I want to see Emerson's final decade not as the destruction
of his philosophies or the undermining of his work, but as their
fulfillment, as a natural extension of his vocation. The man
who claimed to be an endless seeker "with no Past at my back"
was quite literally forgetting his past. The man who, in "Experience," clapped his hands in "infantine joy and amazement,"
relished life's simple pleasures: playing with his grandchildren,
walking outside, visiting with friends. Lidian described him in
this time as the happiest person she ever knew "waking each
morning in a joyful mood." Upon looking at a brilliant red rose
with his poet friend Le Baron Russell, a frail Emerson lifted
his hat and bowed to the rose, saying, "I take off my hat to
it." Decades earlier in "Self-Reliance," he commended roses for
their pure presence: "There is no time to them. There is simply
the rose; it is perfect in every moment of its existence." His life
with dementia, it seems, was marked by the pure presence to
which he so aspired; he possessed "the gift of purely spiritual
continuity," as Howells put it. He who was so given to spontaneity and the following of his own light—"I would write on

the lintels of the door-post, *Whim*"—submitted to the whim of memory loss at the last.

A certain whimsy did seem to accompany Emerson to the end. On one of his late-life evening strolls through Concord, Emerson reportedly looked up toward the starry sky and said to Ellen, "Those things above us, are they not the creation of will?" A question of cosmic import, the pondering of divine agency, a pointed articulation of the universal existential problem: Is creation, are *we*, willed or accidental? Are the stars the work of the deity's half-hid lamp, or wholly without divine attribution? So what is real, what is true? From his question, "it might be inferred that he was meditating on the deepest problem of the universe," writes Robert Underwood Johnson, whose 1923 book *Remembered Yesterdays* contains this anecdote. However, the inquiry was not just what it seemed. Emerson wished to know if the telephone lines overhead, which stretched from pole to pole, were the work of his son-in-law Will, a telephone officer in the region.

7

She Recognizes You

ONE OF MY FIRST MEMORIES OF EVELYN, A RESIDENT AT the Gardens, was on Election Day 2012. She was in her wheelchair watching CNN in the common living room down the hallway from her assisted living apartment. "I will be voting for *that* man," she declared, pointing to Barack Obama on the television screen. She could not recall his name, but she recognized it when I said it. Despite her growing forgetfulness, she insisted on getting to the polls. A former math teacher, she had been the head of her teachers' union, and "a card-carrying Democrat," she said. I appreciated Evelyn's sense of citizenship and pride in her vocation—and how she would, as I mentioned at the beginning of the book, inquire how *my* students were faring.

As her dementia deepened, Evelyn moved from her assisted living apartment to the dementia unit, where she often sat alone, in her wheelchair, by the nurses' station. Sometimes she calmly passed the time, and sometimes she anxiously beseeched passersby. On one midwinter day, when I greeted Evelyn, she asked me to help her get to the street, so she could get home. Her steely blue eyes were wide and urgent. Her shoulders high and tense, she tightly gripped the sides of her wheelchair. She didn't want to keep her mother waiting, she explained. I told her how bitter cold it was outside (and it was) and proposed that we go to her room down the hallway for now, so we could visit. Although she would have preferred my help getting to her mother, she agreed to the suggestion. I walked alongside her as she wheeled her chair down the long hallway.

As we approached her room, I noticed a paper, with ABOUT ME in boldface across the top, posted inside a shadow box on the wall outside her door. The paper contained a photograph of a smiling Evelyn and a few paragraphs about her life. For want of a better idea, I read the sheet aloud. I learned she was born in 1919, which made her ninety-five years old at the time. She was active in her local Catholic parish and grew up in a large, tightly knit Irish family in northern New Jersey. She had never married, and her dearest friend was her cousin Boo. I learned more about her union activity and her long tenure at the high school where she taught. After I finished reading, I looked back to Evelyn, who was staring fixedly into my face, her eyes brimming with tears.

"Thank you," she said. "That makes me feel good." She paused and then opined, "It's lonely when no one knows you."

"Yes, it is lonely sometimes," I said. Recalling her initial intent when I encountered her, I added, "I bet you miss your mother, Evelyn."

"Oh, yes," she responded, emphatically. "Do *you* miss *your* mother?"

In what I can only describe as an act of pure presence, of generous reciprocity, she looked in my eyes and awaited a response. Residents at the nursing home rarely asked me questions, let alone one so emotionally pointed. Usually the question-asker, I seldom offered glimpses into my personal life—a protective position I found comfortable. Evelyn's tender spontaneity, her unguarded curiosity, disarmed me. *Do I miss my mother?* she wanted to know. At the time, I lived a thousand miles from my mom, so I did not see her often. I did, in fact, miss her, which I had never outright admitted to myself or anyone else. After living far from my family for over a decade, I had grown accustomed to distance. Evelyn loosened me from grown-up sophistication, from playing the mature adult who had gained geographical and emotional independence. A lump of sadness pressed against my chest and tightened my throat. She identified an ache within me, one I had not recognized until that moment. This was about me, too.

"Yes, I do," I replied.

Evelyn offered a knowing nod. The source of her urgency and sadness became palpable to me. Imagine: she had not seen her mother for a *very* long time. And no one ever gets over being orphaned, not at any age. No one stops searching for home or for her mother.

My conversation with Evelyn was not just what it seemed; it was not simply a woman confused about the year and the whereabouts of her long-deceased mother. I recognized something deeper in her yearning; she recognized something hidden in me.

More than other conditions, dementia raises questions of what it means to know—the self, another. A person's ability to recognize—usually defined as the capacity to properly identify the name and role of another—emerges as a supreme anxiety surrounding dementia. I have witnessed how distraught relatives and friends have become when their loved ones called them by the wrong name (or no name) or mistook them as, say, their mother instead of their daughter. I recall a husband asking his wife to identify each person in a family photo he held before her. When she hesitated, he would plead, "You know who that is. Don't you remember?"

An incident at a lecture I attended some years back at Furman University revealed to me some of the cultural and emotional stock we place in recognition. The speaker was the director of some major environmental organization. He obviously loved the material and felt passionately about his work, but there was a problem. Even though he stood, flanked by huge purple banners bearing Furman's logo, before a room full of students sporting all manner of Furman T-shirts, and was warmly welcomed to *Furman* University by administrators and faculty—for his entire lecture, he referred to how wonderful it was to be speaking at *Elon* University to a room full of Elon students and faculty, how he had enjoyed earlier that day attending a class at Elon, and how much potential this beautiful university, Elon, had.

At first, I felt embarrassed for him. Surely, this was a slip of tongue. Surely, he traveled and spoke so much that, at times, it could be tiring and disorienting. Surely, he would right the ship. But the hour-long lecture continued, and he continued wrongly addressing the room. At the first couple of mentions of Elon, the room squirmed uncomfortably, a few giggles escaped. As the misnaming continued, the mood of the gathering shifted to frustration and then to disengagement with the speaker. My friend, a Furman professor, shifted uncomfortably in his chair, and let out exasperated sighs. Soon, my own embarrassment *for* the speaker turned to anger *at* him. *How much is this guy getting paid again? I mean, doesn't he see who is right before him? How sloppy and inattentive can you be? How terribly rude!*

This relatively innocuous story—no one was harmed by being mistaken for Elon students—reminds me how closely we associate the ability to name and the capacity to care. Our own sense of worth is tied up in other people knowing and speaking our names. And we harshly judge those who fail to recognize us after they have what we believe is sufficient exposure to us. We link their forgetting to self-centeredness or lack of concern—and, in turn, we believe we do not owe them our attention and concern. The Q&A portion of the lecture was short and unenthusiastic, as students and faculty alike seemed to possess little interest in further engaging the speaker.

While some forms of nonrecognition or misrecognition *do* stem from aloofness, other forms, of course, do not. But it is hard to shake the heavy judgments and negative visceral reactions, even when we know that the limits of someone's brain prevent certain types of recall. We seem to forget that *lack* of care is possible despite someone's ability to "recognize" us—and, conversely, care is possible apart from precise naming. The medical anthropologist Janelle Taylor, in her 2008 article "On Recognition, Caring, and Dementia," explores the sources and implications of this anxiety over recognition. She writes what she calls an "autoethnographic" account of her experiences as a daughter to a mother with Alzheimer's disease. Taylor notes that when friends, colleagues, and acquaintances first learn about her mother's dementia, they always ask some form of the same question: *Does she recognize you?*

Not only does Taylor find the question difficult to answer and increasingly irrelevant, she wonders why this particular question is so ubiquitous. "She may not 'recognize' me in a narrowly cognitive sense," Taylor writes, "but my Mom does 'recognize' me as someone who is there with her, someone familiar perhaps, and she does not need to have all the details sorted out in order to 'care' for me." When many people ask

the same question over and over again, Taylor's anthropology
training tells her, it probably indicates "something important
and unresolved about social life." Taylor suspects that another
question lurks behind the seemingly innocent curiosity about
her mother's ability to recognize her: "Do you, do *we*, recognize
her? Do we *grant her recognition*?" Whether or not her mother is
deemed worthy of the same civic, collective responsibility af-
forded to others seems to hinge on the manifestation of a particular cognitive ability. Only if she is able to recognize others
is she a candidate for greater social recognition.

Taylor pinpoints a dynamic that I, too, have witnessed *ad
nauseam* with respect to people with dementia: "[O]ften other
people stop 'recognizing' and 'caring' about *them*." One's ability
to recognize seems to serve as a litmus test for personhood.
With only one exception, none of Taylor's mother's many
friends visit her after she moves into a care facility, despite
Taylor's invitations. Although warm and kind individually, as
a group they abandon her. It's the threat of social death I've
mentioned before. On top of physical and mental losses, persons with dementia often suffer social losses.

I suspect that Taylor's mother, my grandfather, the residents
at the Gardens are at risk for social erasure because they show
signs of yielding to the same forces that we know will eventually overcome each one of us. Hoping to avoid the normalcy
of death and its discomforting realities (especially mental demise), we push away their representatives. Largely implicit, this
dynamic arises, not because we naïvely believe dementia won't

ever happen to us, but because we sense that it might—that, in fact, it *will*.

When Mum was still Mum. I came across the phrase some years back in an essay whose writer used it to refer to her mother before Alzheimer's. I wrote it down in my journal, finding it strange to refer to someone who is still living as existing in past tense. I have since forgotten which magazine and which author. It doesn't matter, I suppose, mostly because the phrase no longer strikes me as exceptional or worthy of specific citation. After coming upon innumerable variations on it, I recognize it now as common dementia shorthand, more cliché than oddity. *Back when so-and-so was still so-and-so* characterizes persons before their advancing dementia, with the gut-punch of the implied, tragic corollary: Janie is no longer Janie; Mum is no longer Mum; Person is no longer Person.

The sentiment speaks to the disorienting discontinuities and ruptured relationships that often accompany dementia. The speaker grasps for language to express the real pain of intimate grief. Nevertheless, I am wary of the assumptions behind it, wary of a dubious confidence in one's ability to accurately judge when the person is no longer the person—or to completely know or have known the person in the first place. The grammatical trope reflects a cultural dogma: the *real* person is the pre-dementia person. A person's identity can and should remain relatively stable across time and space, so when significant and even jarring changes occur, the person with dementia becomes a lesser, falser version of a once-full, real human being. She is presumed to have little or no continuity with the pre-dementia person. She can offer nothing revelatory or insightful about her past or present identity. Thus, she is no longer recognized as the "real" Mum. Our language reveals the propensity to deny persons with dementia full recognition.

But recognition is not unidirectional; it's no one-way street. Steven Sabat's idea of "social personae" helped me reframe my approach to persons with dementia and take responsibility for the part I play in recognizing another. An important manifestation of personal identity, one's "social personae" require the cooperation of others in the social world. A teacher needs students to acknowledge her as such; a loving spouse needs a partner to support this role. Persons with dementia are especially vulnerable to having valued social aspects of their selfhood undermined, as others define them primarily by their deficits. They are seen as disease sufferers, confused patients, passive victims, while cherished, long-standing roles, such as loyal friend, involved parent, dutiful worker, are no longer readily recognized or supported.

By taking attempts at communication seriously, we respect the many possible dimensions that persons may seek to express—through and despite the limits of their illness. When Evelyn expressed worry about her long-dead mother, perhaps she was more a Devoted Daughter than a Perseverating Patient. The role assigned to her will determine the response to her. A Perseverating Patient's concern is a disease symptom; it marks confusion. A Devoted Daughter's concern is legitimate; it makes sense. It is not a matter of denying the fact of impairment and its real challenges, but it is to declare that defect is not the whole story.

My friend Nancy's dad spent his professional life as a church pastor and hospital chaplain. He lived his final years with dementia at an assisted living facility. One of his neighbors at the facility developed cancer and soon began to receive hospice care. Late at night, Nancy's dad, using his walker, would make his way down the hallway and enter the woman's room. He sat beside her bed and talked to her (even though she could not talk back) and softly touched her hand. Nancy first learned of her father's nighttime visits to this dying woman at his funeral, from the woman's friend. "He had no memory of being a preacher," Nancy told me, "but he was still ministering."

Long after my grandfather retired from medicine—and deep into his dementia—he was still practicing, too. He kept an attentive eye on the well-being of other nursing home residents, sometimes pushing wheelchairs or guiding walkers—and even making occasional comments that revealed his clinical concern. On one occasion right after Jack had moved from his house to a care facility, he had tried to help another resident stand after she had fallen. Staff members wrongly assumed he was "attacking" the resident and rushed to pull him away from her, ordering him to let her go. They had misrecognized him, reflexively assigning him the negative role of Belligerent

Patient, until my mother corrected them: he's the Attending Physician. They began to call him "Dr. Jack" and thank him for his assistance. If the staff had prevented Nancy's dad from offering gestures of care or had continued to misunderstand my grandfather's actions as aberrant, they would have denied them cherished roles and denied others their kindnesses. They would have ushered in a kind of social death.

The question of recognition is not just what it seems. It throws into new relief the old problem of bodies. Dementia highlights and troubles the propensity to separate the mind from the body, and to idealize and dematerialize the former. The confused language around dementia—*his mind is going, but his body is still strong*; *the body "outlasts" the brain*—suggests one's mind or brain exists apart from one's body, which places dementia outside the body's ordinary functions and afflictions. If dementia is a damaged mind, and the mind is synonymous with spirit, soul, self, then dementia takes on an extraordinary moral charge. *Does she recognize you?*—an apparent prying into certain capacities of the body's brain—becomes a quasi-spiritual inquiry into the status of one's very self.

I turn to Nancy Mairs's book *Carnal Acts* for help unraveling this mind/body split—a dualism that makes dementia into a robber of selves, souls, essential identities. Reflecting on her life with multiple sclerosis, Mairs likens her experience with the disease's erratic symptoms to being "haunted by a capricious and mean-spirited ghost," who trips her, squeezes her bladder, and overcomes her with fatigue. "An alien invader must be at work," she writes. "But of course it's not. It's your own body. That is, it's you." Living with a degenerative neurological disease leads Mairs to an inescapable awareness of her body. Her condition, she declares, has "rammed my 'self' straight back into the body I had been trained to believe it could, through high-minded acts and aspirations, rise above."

Mairs challenges the Western tradition that separates the mind from the body, the self from the flesh. This same tradition associates the male with the mind, and the female with the flesh. This split, she reminds us, is not a benign pairing of complementary equals. Separate is never equal. Rather, bodies are treated much the same as women, as "subordinates, inferior in moral status." Amid forces that seek to suppress robust moral accountings of the body, especially women's bodies, Mairs claims the power of her voice as emerging from her crippled body. She refuses to succumb to shame, refuses to remain silent. Recognizing the inseparability of communication—in her case, writing—from the flesh that produces it, Mairs asserts, "No body, no voice; no voice, no body. That's what I know in my bones."

Like MS, dementia bears the burdens of the mind-body hierarchy. Dementia, too, entails brain damage, and we have imagined the brain and its workings as separate from the body—as the ephemeral and superior "mind." The mind, after all, is *supposed* to "rise above" the body. When we come face to face with the brain's degeneration, we are reminded of its inseparability from the rest of our mutable flesh. Dementia rams the mind back into the body, reminding us that it has been there all along, right under—or, more precisely, *behind*—our noses. Previously imagined as free, transcending the carnal and mundane, acting objectively (and thus morally) without bodily encumbrance, the mind reigned over the body, subordinating its unruly and base desires. Dementia reveals the mind as inextricably bound to the utterly corruptible brain, to bodily gray matter. The imperishable has put on the perishable—*has always had it on*. And discursively, if the mind is male and the body is female, then when the mind is laid bare as embodied, when it is revealed as flesh, the mind turns feminine; it suffers emasculation. Dementia rips the veil, exposing the illusory male as intrinsically female. By patriarchal logic, this switch signals a terrible demotion: the pollution and denigration of the mind. The assumption that men—namely, *white* men—are closely aligned with reason and rationality, the supposed "higher" forms of being, relegates women, men of color, and nonbinary people to the "lower" realms of the flesh.

This position and its dubious logic demand serious revision. The mind's return to the body need not portend failure. If we take a broad view of the body, then what we call the mind both encompasses and transcends the workings of a solitary brain. The mind is freed to exist within a larger unity, within a complex, whole organism irreducible to isolate parts. Inextricably related to other bodies, the mind joins a dynamic, robust ecosystem. No piece exists in isolation from or in domination over another. Grounded in the concrete, the mind is no longer opposed to the body—no longer its distant ruler, its harsh disciplinarian, its persnickety landlord. When the head weakens, it does not indicate a globally failed state. There is no antagonism between mind and body because there is no superiority. There is no superiority because there is no independent existence.

Although my own faith tradition has often perpetuated a damaging mind/body duality, I find early teachings regarding the resurrection—in which transcendence comes through the body, not apart from or despite it—a source of hope. Rather than a necessary but disappointing warehouse for the spirit, the body is a temple. The Apostles' Creed's *I believe in the resurrection of the body* forces confessors to admit (eagerly, reluctantly, vacantly?) an eccentric, even creepy, fleshiness. This creedal declaration takes its cue from Gospel accounts of a bodily post-resurrection Jesus, who eats fish, breaks bread, and cooks breakfast. He breathes on the disciples. His hands, feet, and side bear scars. He sits, stands, walks, and talks. In John's Gospel, Mary Magdalene hugs him, wrapping her arms around a real body. Although Jesus's resurrected body is different from regular flesh—he walks through doors, he appears and disappears suddenly, his fatal wounds have healed into scars—all of the Gospel writers seem clear: the post-resurrection Jesus is not immaterial.

The resurrection of Jesus's body locates transcendence in hemoglobin and leukocytes, in salivary glands and the distal gut, in neurons and dendrites, in mushy, mutable flesh. Perhaps even more preposterous than a belief in the resurrection of *his* body, believers profess the resurrection of *the* body. *Our* pulpy innards, porous bones, prefrontal cortices, pocked cheeks are all coming back, too, it seems. In this way, Christian ortho- doxy proves squarely and unbelievably weird. And I appreciate its implications for dementia, which carries its own embodied peculiarities. This matter of resurrection grounds believers deeper and deeper in physicality—"in bone and blood" and "the pulse in the wound," writes the mystic poet Denise Lever- tov. But the resurrection resolves nothing, other than blowing to pieces any insistence on mind over body, spirit over flesh. No body, no resurrection. No resurrection, no body. That's what I know in my bones.

When the body becomes the site of redemption, and the mind does not escape the body, a certain unity can abide. The matter of recognition gets fleshed out. No longer does demen- tia have to bear an extraordinary moral burden. No longer does a memory deficit indicate a deficient mind, soul, spirit. No longer does a blemished brain indicate a defective self that gradually and hopelessly vacates its body. The brain, in all its vagaries, remains part of the body, which is no less a temple, no less the source of hope and resurrection because of its wounds. The onus of recognition moves beyond the capabilities of one body's discrete brain. Shattering notions of self-containment, of narrow definitions of *knowing*, dementia refuses the abstrac- tion of straight lines, including any neat border between flesh and spirit, body and mind. The circle of what it means to know and be known widens, rushing outward to new and larger circles—which strikes me as good news, before and after I have dementia.

In *First Cousin Once Removed*, the director Alan Berliner probes the poet Edwin Honig, his cousin, for what he can still remember, asking him repeatedly throughout the film variations on the question, "Do you know who I am?" While I understand the filmmaker's curiosity, it now strikes me that asking someone who has trouble thinking to recall something is the equivalent of asking someone who has a dislocated shoulder to lift something. Halfway through the film, Honig—whom I suspect is tired of being made the fool—reverses the question, asking Berliner, "Do you know who you are?" A brief silence ensues; the film jump-cuts to Berliner's face in profile as he listens to Honig play seemingly random notes on a piano. Perhaps, persons with dementia call us to confront our own ambiguity, to realize just how difficult it is to pin down one's own identity, let alone someone else's. My friend Janet's mother, in the depths of dementia, asked her one day, "Are you me?" Janet hesitated. *Well, not exactly. But, yes, sort of.* Possessing knowledge of one's self and others is not a dilemma just for those deep in dementia; it is a human quandary.

"What is a man anyhow? what am I? what are you?" asks Whitman in "Song of Myself." The self-proclaimed poet of the body and poet of the soul tries on, extends, experiments, expands. Turning around and around questions of identity, he comes to no fast or fixed conclusions. Whitman invites readers to imagine and reimagine the self as wide, contradictory, and multitudinous. Obfuscation marks selfhood: "I too am not a bit tamed, I too am untranslatable." This wildly broad self is never disembodied, never a neutered omniscience, but rather lives and moves within a wide circulation of bodies. While maintaining the specific magnificence of his own body—"the narrowest hinge in my hand puts to scorn all machinery"—Whitman declares he is "part of every other body" and "not contain'd between my hat and boots."

Three centuries before Whitman, Michel de Montaigne observed the range of variation within individuals. Even that which *seems* contained between "hat and boots"—the intricacies of any one body—resists discrete, uniform accounting. "We are entirely made up of bits and pieces, woven together so diversely and so shapelessly that each of them pulls its own way at every moment," writes Montaigne. When I read his essays, his attempts at self-understanding, I get the sense that Montaigne knows the diversity of which he speaks. His reflections run the gamut from seemingly juvenile observations about flatulence and erections, to stunning sensitivities about intimate love and dying well. "[A]nyone who turns his prime attention on to himself," Montaigne asserts, "will hardly ever find himself in the same state twice." Multiplicity marks us and makes us. Rather than a seamless, uniform piece, each of us is an irregular tapestry, shapeless and diverse—each garment, its own unique assemblage of "bits and pieces."

Choice and circumstance, biology and geography, history, luck and grace, tangle to create this discrete garment—what I call *me* and *you*. Hardly in the same state twice, hardly fixed, we remain shapeless, diverse, pulled. Perhaps we are not so much entirely amorphous as our patterns are difficult and scrappy—always constituting and constituted by vaster tapestries.

One reviewer of *First Cousin Once Removed* said the film made it hard to answer the question "When did Honig stop being Honig?" Perhaps the question was hard to answer because it presumed that he did, in fact, stop being himself—and that any of us can entirely cease being ourselves. Rather, as certain facets of ourselves fade or seemingly vanish, other qualities remain and still others may emerge or grow more prominent. That only or primarily negative traits surface in dementia is a popular trope: the gentle person who turns violent; the mild-mannered man who now spews obscenities. But this narrative is partial. Janelle Taylor finds her mother "the cheerful, affectionate person" she has always known, who even helps Taylor to "slow down enough to gain a new appreciation of the moment." While she acknowledges that the experiences of other families may be far more negative than hers, Taylor asserts, "[M]y mother's dementia is no 'horror story'—and this, too, lies within the domain of the possible." My relationship with my grandfather in his later years was no "horror story" either, as a certain calm connection grew between us.

I recently listened to a podcast on Safe Space Radio that featured the "untold stories of dementia"; in one of these stories, a woman tells of being on the phone with her father and hearing her mother in the background say, "My daughter? Oh, I *love* her." The daughter comments, "And she never would've said anything like that ever. My mom had had a harsh life [. . .] And this sweetness that came out when she started to become ill was a lovely surprise." Something harsh was falling away, and something softer was emerging.

The dementia activist and author Kate Swaffer talks about the surprising clarity dementia brought to her life. When I had the chance to meet Swaffer, who lives in Australia, "face to face" via video chat, she told me that when she was first diagnosed with younger-onset dementia, she thought of her world in terms of loss and disappearance. Now she understands that, while the life she once knew before her dementia *has* disappeared, disappearance was and is not the end of her story. "I became a different Kate, not a better or worse Kate," she commented. After a process of grieving and coming to accept "that the old Kate was gone forever," she saw a new world emerging. She said she now sees dementia as a gift, which has helped her to understand "otherness," increasing her empathy for those who endure discrimination. It has shown her who her true friends are and given her renewed purpose as she seeks to change the negative narratives and policies around dementia. "Dementia is full of paradoxes," she asserted. "I know so much more than I did before."

In *In the Shadow of Memory*, Floyd Skoot describes the complex ways in which the changes of his intellectual and emotional experiences interacted "to demand and create a fresh experience of being in the world, an encounter that feels spiritual in nature." Even as Skloot endured the pain of intellectual diminishment, he discovered a new freedom to express his emotions. "Love and passion entered my life for the first time in decades," he writes. His relationship with his daughter deepened, and he renewed a relationship with his terminally ill, estranged brother. While cognitive change does not always hold such happy surprises, such stories offer a counterweight to more dire depictions of dementia; threads of affection, tenderness, and peace are also possible.

Reflecting on the reordering dementia wrought in his life, Skloot declares, "I have been rewoven." Rewoven—placed back on the loom—the bits and pieces of his life get pulled in a new direction, forming a new shape. I have not yet faced such a radical remaking, or the disappearance of one world and the reemergence of another in the way Swaffer described. Nevertheless, I am attempting to reckon now with my own variations, negotiations, and renegotiations, my own bits and pieces, shapeless and pulling. On my way to dementia, I am already living in the fray of a heterogeneous self. On some days, I resonate with the Apostle Paul's admission: "I do not understand my own actions. For I do not do what I want, but I do the very thing I hate." And sometimes I do not know what I want, or which *I* wants what. Each tugs its own way. Perhaps, with some luck, my tatters will get reassembled in a way that produces greater love and passion, a lovely surprise or two.

Memory, it seems, is suspended in the tragic, bound by the collection of trace sensitivities we call intuition, hooked to senses and the resolute living and dying of bodies, held narrowly in the lurch of incalculable desire. It is a kind of summoning that surpasses the storage and retrieval of discrete facts by an individual brain. Memory is lodged in the gut, I think. Perhaps this is what Emerson means when he says, "[O]nly what the affection animates can be remembered." Perhaps, to carefully regard and cultivate our affections now—especially love—might edify the body of a grander remembering, nurturing a broader sense of what it means to recognize.

When we lived in a walk-up apartment, Ryan said he could distinguish my gait, my distinct way of entering the building, my feet on the steps up to our place. He said he always knew when it was me and not one of the similarly weighted women who lived in the apartment across the hall. I asked how, how do you know, how can you tell? He could not explain it, and yet I knew how, even before I asked him. I have recognized him in this way, too, and I could not explain it myself. The rhythm of how he opens and shuts a car door, a kitchen cabinet; the cadence of his breath when he is sleeping; his distinct radiation of heat; the way his body measures distance; the shade of his skin when he is sad; his smell.

Sometimes, when he leaves early in the morning, half-asleep still, I put my face in his pillow and inhale—trying to assume his alluvial traces. Yet I rise to find I cannot capture a body, not even in words, and if not in words, then what? Where does a corpus of memory go? What terrific impermanence: to inhale is to exhale, to remember is to forget. Perhaps what remains is without name, an unsaid word—this memory of the affections, of the gut.

Five years after my grandmother's death, I finally opened the box that contained the dishes she had left to me. They were wrapped in her cloth dinner napkins, silk neck scarves, pocket handkerchiefs, and sewing scraps. The dishes had been thus swathed, cushioned by the material emptied from her drawers, for half a decade—waiting somewhere for me, in my mother's basement.

A smell, so unmistakable and indescribable, emerged from the opened box. It was her house: windowsill herbs and old carpet, heavy drapery and real wood furniture, hard well water and Palmolive Gold bar soap, and dust, loose and floating, in streaming light. It was the scent of palpable gentleness, of slow summer days in her cool, dark den and her low voice reading Little Golden Books to my cousins and me. It also smelled distinctly of moth balls, which my grandmother used liberally for their power to protect and preserve. This faint but familiar stench betrayed her conserving impulse; she guarded and saved every jot and tittle no matter its worth. This inclination gave way to a certain unyielding miserliness, which, I admit, I hated. Still, I loved her and admired how little she discarded in an era of utter waste.

An instant as ordinary as opening a box and inhaling can quicken the psyche—a reminder that as long as we breathe on this seething planet, as long as we feel, we cannot be free from remembering.

During Holy Week, Sister Donna, the nun with whom I worked at the nursing home, offered an annual Maundy Thursday service for the residents, and she invited me, the interfaith chaplain, to participate. The service occurred in the Gardens' largest space, a multifunction room with industrial-grade gray carpet, a small kitchenette in the back corner, and a wall of windows that looked out onto a garden. Peel-off seasonal decals (butterflies and daffodils for spring) decorated the room's windows, obscuring the view of the actual outdoors. The sixty or so residents who attended, most of whom sat in wheelchairs, were placed in neat rows that spanned the length of the room.

From a small lectern, Sister read the scripture lesson from John's Gospel. After Jesus washes his disciples' feet on the night before his death, he gives them a new commandment ("Maundy," I learned lately, is from the Latin for "mandate" or "commandment"). Sister slowed, allowing the weight of the mandate to fall upon its hearers: "A new command I give you: Love one another. As I have loved you, so you must love one another." After the reading, she approached the portable altar—a wooden box on wheels, covered by a tablecloth—and picked up a small etched-glass pitcher. She entered the rows of residents and slowly poured water over each person's open palms—a modified "foot washing." I stood beside her, stooping forward with a small bowl in my hands to catch the runoff.

On my final Holy Week at the Gardens, this service, which had always struck me as powerful, took on an additional charge because of Victoria, a resident who had moved to the facility in recent months. She was tall and sturdy, with an easy smile and high, chirpy voice. She regularly attended the small group Bible studies I facilitated on her assisted living floor. Often chiming into the discussion, she offered what seemed like a jumble of half-sentences. Her genial affect and tone of voice suggested her approval, a friendly sentiment of some sort—even though I rarely made sense of the content of her comments. I appreciated Victoria's affable presence in the group but felt somewhat embarrassed when she spoke. Because I knew her only in this setting, Victoria seemed pleasantly confused to me. While I intended no particular disrespect to Victoria, my automatic evaluation of her was unimaginative, facile, careless, institutional.

The "pleasantly confused" are an institution's model dementia patients: compliant, redirectable, sweetly docile. Operational ease and efficiency drive large nursing facilities, and the pleasantly confused conform nicely to this schema. They present no resistance. A frictionless environment—keeping pleasant people pleasant and turning agitated people pleasant—emerges as the institutional ideal, often at the expense of supporting individual complexities. A pleasant life does not necessarily translate into a meaningful life. Even as individual workers and innovative programs seek to buck the trend, the dominant setup incentivizes a well-ordered classroom, a tyranny of the calm. Beholden to bottom lines and forced to exist *en masse* by an ageist society, these facilities are charged with an inhumanly gargantuan task. With 180 residents in my care, some of whom were transparently distressed, I was happy to find a resident pleasant, confused, and nothing more. Even so, I was not, am not, excused from a greater mandate. Holy Thursday gave me a chance to look again.

Sister approached Victoria and extended her palms to show her what to do. Victoria mirrored her, cupping her hands. I bent forward with the bowl as Sister Donna poured the water and offered a blessing: "May God's Spirit refresh you. May you know Jesus's unconditional love and share this love with all those you meet." As the water covered Victoria's hands, I observed her face transform from what I had deemed benign but unfocused—to utter, intent attention. Her features slackened and broadened. Tense lines around her eyes softened, lines I had never noticed until they disappeared. Her cheeks flushed, and her strong frame shook, as she began to softly weep. Her sobs sprung from a center: tender, solid, and sure.

For once, I saw her roundly, as a person in dynamic motion, circling an ineffable cause. Victoria drew me within the orbit of her exquisite core, and spun me back out again, converted. I saw beyond my surface vision. The air cleared, and the clouds lifted a little, apprising me of a new and excellent region of life—hers, mine. In my small vessel, I received the streams that ran from her flesh.

"She remembered all of who she is," Sister commented to me after the service, with her usual spiritual astuteness. I remembered, too.

In my search for new, more robust renderings of dementia, I return to an ancient rumination on memory—Book X of Augustine's *Confessions*. Augustine scrupulously probes his memory, searching for God therein. "But whereabouts in my memory do you dwell, Lord, in which part of it do you abide?" he pleads. Pursuing the answer, Augustine scrutinizes his storehouse of memories, classifying and collecting his thoughts, searching for the whereabouts of truth, of the divine. He investigates everything, from how he can recall emotions without directly feeling them in the act of remembering, to how he can remember forgetfulness, to how he can remember God if God isn't already planted in his memory.

Encountering at once the majesty and the limits of his memories, Augustine admits, "No single one of them could I have perceived without you, but I found that no single one of them was you." His thoughts, he observes, emerge from a process in which the scattered and disordered memories within him are pulled up from "distant caverns" and "herded together."

Scattered memories are "collected again," which is why, Augustine notes, the mind has properly claimed the verb "cogitate"—root *cogo*, or "to collect"—for this activity of thought.

By Book X's end, Augustine determines, "Nowhere amid all these things which I survey under your guidance do I find a safe haven for my soul except in you; only there are the *scattered elements of my being collected* [emphasis added], so that no part of me may escape from you." God—and not Augustine's personal capacity for memory, however formidable—emerges as the ultimate recollector, cogitator, recognizer. Only in the refuge of the divine memory is what is scattered gathered, what is lost found. No fragment, scrap, or crumb escapes holy cover. The Augustine who famously declared, "I have become a vast enigma to myself," seems to find a certain rest in the vast enigma of divine memory. I feel some relief, too. If a Holy Other collects all of what is scattered and lost, then I suppose I don't have to keep it all together.

"I don't know who I am anymore," Anthea confided in me on the first visit I made to her and Fred, her wheelchair-bound husband and caregiver, after they had moved to an assisted living apartment in the Gardens. When Fred overheard her admission, he quickly corrected his wife, voiding her claim: "You do too!" He proceeded to quiz her on the names of their children. I believed Anthea. She felt she was falling to pieces and no longer sensed herself as an abiding whole. Not long after this visit, Fred became unable to care for Anthea, so she was moved to the dementia unit.

A devout Lutheran who had worked as her church's secretary, Anthea began attending the floor's small prayer group, composed entirely of women. In slow, deliberate, sorrowful speech, she shared with the group on her first day: "The doctor told me . . . I forget a lot of things." Mary, the group stalwart who had declared how blessed she must be for not having it all together, responded, "That's okay. We all forget things. The person you're talking to probably forgets, too." Rose, who sat in a special reclining wheelchair and rarely spoke, added, "Oh yes! I think it's good to forget some things. You don't have to always remember. It's like having a blank slate!" The survivor of an abusive marriage, Rose perhaps benefited more than most from the relief of having a "blank slate." When Bernice nodded in agreement, I thought of her blank slate, too. When I first met her, she was giving bags of shoes to male staff members—a strange behavior made grim by the fact that these were the shoes of her husband, who had died a few days before. She was also suffering from paranoid delusions about being pregnant. As her dementia progressed, some of the anguish associated with her long-standing mental illness seemed to subside. She seemed lighter, quicker to laugh and less prone to disconnect from her present reality.

In that moment, the group recognized Anthea. They recognized her struggle as their struggle. Sometimes the pieces get picked up, the threads get returned to the loom and rewoven, by astonishing, unlikely recollectors. When I was with these women, a peculiar yet hopeful notion sometimes occurred to me: when dementia changes my brain, might I grow closer to the divine, whose ways are not your ways, whose thoughts are not your thoughts?

"You came to see me!"

Carol's spry greeting surprised me as I stepped into her room and sat in the chair next to her bed. She was sitting up, smiling. I was not used to such effervescence in these times. Carol was on hospice and all signs indicated that her death was near. She was gaunt, having taken only small sips of fluids in recent days. Her skin had grown pallid, and she slept most of the day.

"Oh, it is just so good to see you, Terry! It has been so long," she exclaimed, her eyes alight, wide and clear-peering. "I thought you'd *never* come."

She gazed tenderly into my face, as if I were not the chaplain she had just met in recent weeks, as if she and I shared a long and wondrous history together. Carol recognized me as Terry, likely a long-dead relative or friend, which is likely why it had been so long. I squirmed. I was new enough to the work that I worried she might realize that I was not Terry and become sad or angry. This is the terribly literalistic thinking of people who are not imminently dying.

We have no idea the great many meanings of our presence,

the great many manifestations we bring. We simply show up, loose and floating, within a field, mostly not of our own making. Sometimes we are recognized, but not as whom we take ourselves to be. We can resist and dismiss this "misrecognition" as unfounded projection, or we can embrace it as somehow revealing aspects of ourselves, however obscure to ourselves.

Terry was a stranger to me but not to Carol. In this instance, my presence sparked gladness. I have also sparked sadness, anger, fear. I still can hear the end-stage cancer patient who cried out when I entered his room: "Not you! No! I don't want you!" I contain joy, fear, anger, sadness, so why would I not have the power to elicit these emotions in others? I try to take neither welcome nor rejection exceptionally personally (or impersonally).

"Hello, Carol. I'm glad to see you, too," I said.

We held hands. We did not say much. She seemed content to look upon Terry's face, my face. She drifted to sleep and died a few days later.

8

When I Have Dementia

"I HOPE YOU'LL STILL LAUGH AT MY JOKES WHEN I HAVE dementia," I said to Ryan on an evening walk not long after my thirty-fourth birthday. It was the first time I had tried out my new resolution to stop saying "*if* I get dementia" and to start referring to the time "*when* I have dementia." I felt the catch in my throat, a node of reluctance, but I was committed now. I had heard of this turn of phrase from a fifty-something nursing home administrator who said she uses "when I have dementia" to reflect a calculation of her odds, given her particular family history and the fact that mental decline is probable as we age. I appreciated her tough-minded devotion to naming her probabilities, and I thought I would adopt this practice, too.

At that time, Jack was living in the Veterans Home, entering what I now know were the final months of his life. And I had just learned that his dad, my maternal great-grandfather, had exhibited the same sort of progressive forgetfulness in his old age. My paternal grandfather had died from cancer at seventy and one of his brothers had been killed in WWII, but I wondered about the fate of his other siblings. I dug out my copy of *Casteel Cousins*, a thin, spiral-bound family history written by a genealogist cousin, and uncovered the ubiquity of dementia:

> Esther's mind, which had been so competently organized and managed everything, was fading.

> In Bobby's last few years, the gradual and terrible debilitations of Alzheimer's disease forced her to withdraw, first, to a homebound existence, and then to a dependent life in a specialized care facility.

> Apparently he had Alzheimer's disease which has afflicted other members of the family. Being physically strong, Richard survived for several years but eventually this disease caused his death.

I returned the booklet to its storage bin; I do not recall feeling much of anything, perhaps only a faint sense of resignation. There was not much I could do with this new information.

Three years later, in 2017, as I was close to completing a draft of this book, *The New York Times* ran the article "What If You Knew Alzheimer's Was Coming for You?" A friend, knowing of my project, sent it to me. The article talks about ApoE4, a variant of the protein-regulating ApoE gene that increases the risk of Alzheimer's, and an online support group that has formed for people who possess the variant. I had heard of an "Alzheimer's gene" associated with late-onset dementia, but I had not thought much about it, mostly because I have resisted reducing dementia discourse to strictly clinical or deterministic terms. The fearful image, suggested by the article's title, of Alzheimer's as a predator coming for its prey was exactly the kind of metaphor I was hoping to undermine. But I suppose I was not immune to the power of dread-inducing reductions, after all; the article piqued my interest—*was* Alzheimer's coming for me?

Earlier that year, my parents had undergone a battery of genetic testing, and my mom had emailed me their results. Given my history of migraines, she was concerned about a possible blood-clotting mutation I may have inherited. After reading the *Times* article, I wondered if those results also had contained their ApoE profile. After a tedious search through my inbox, I found her message, which bore the vague subject line "3 Pages"; the body contained no text. The three attached documents were scanned lab reports, out of focus and cut off at the bottom. Nevertheless, I thought I saw that both of my parents carried one copy of ApoE4. I emailed my mom, and she quickly confirmed my findings. Nearly five hours after her initial response, she sent a follow-up message, just after midnight, expressing her worry that I would "advertise" her and my dad's genetics in my book. She recommended that I get myself tested, or "at least wait until we are demented," she half-joked. My mother rarely stays up past 10:00 p.m. unless something is keeping her up; I suspected, with some guilt, that my inquiry had worried her, disrupting her nighttime routine. I replied, "I could do the test . . . a good idea."

Apparently, I could pay $199, spit into a tube, and gain the results of my genotype in six to eight weeks. It was that easy. Of course, revealing my genes would, in part, "advertise" my parents' genes—I suppose I am already a walking advertisement— but I understood my mother's concern (and have since received their permission). The *Times* article reports that many of the members of the ApoE4 support group, some of whom carry only one copy of the gene, wish to remain anonymous for fear of being denied insurance—in addition to general worries over social stigma.

For weeks, I waffled on whether to take the test. Was it, in fact, ". . . a good idea"? Sometimes I felt sure I should take it, reasoning that resolving doubt is brave, and knowledge can be power. And sometimes I hedged, reasoning that preserving uncertainty is humble, and certain knowledge can be a burden.

In my less high-minded moments, I imagined what a good "hook" it would be for the book if I had one or two copies of ApoE4—dramatically upping my personal stake. I also fantasized about how I would stage my sense of relief if I discovered that I possessed no copies.

I ultimately decided not to take the test, to live only with my probabilities—at least for the time being. My interest in dementia has never risen or fallen on personal risk and lab tests, I reminded myself. The habitual routing of all things "dementia" back to the clinical, diagnostic, and prognostic is what I am hoping to avoid anyway. Or maybe I am just too scared to know. Whatever the case, I am convinced that preparing for and preventing disorder—skills that in other areas of life have served me well—can only take me so far with dementia. Preparing for dementia requires me to hone other abilities, such as embracing spontaneity and ambiguity, and nurturing friendships beyond convenience—which feel like important endeavors no matter one's genetic code. And finding out my profile for the sake of adding a possible dramatic component to the book seemed not only unkind to myself but also distracting from my larger points. The subject is mortality, and no tube of spit can entirely predict its course or prepare its "sufferers."

The allure of knowing does not wholly subside, however. I consider my incomparable grandfather, no longer keeping score. I consider the women on the dementia unit, rising to prayer. I consider my grandfather's fiery sisters, each forgetting in her turn. Beyond all reason, I have loved my brain. I mourn the foot pressing down upon the skull. A genetic risk factor does not determine one's fate, I understand. Nevertheless, I have no reason to believe I am exceptional or lucky. I do not believe in cures. I do not believe I will be spared.

My syntactical conversion from *if* to *when* began before I knew my parents' genotype and my statistical realities. This new knowledge perhaps further solidified the switch. But, more than an interest in my personal probabilities, I am animated by the desire to close the psychological distance between those who have dementia *now* ("them") and those who do not have dementia *yet* ("us"). My revised language reflects a larger life project to embrace people who have dementia, to deconstruct negative and stigmatizing attitudes toward brain disease, and to construct a more excellent way through dementia's snares. It reminds me that dementia is the story I am inside, now—quite literally, given my family history and professional commitments, but also in a broader, harder-to-define spiritual sense.

I choose to incorporate "when I have dementia" into my lexicon, which means I have a choice not to, which means I still hold a privileged distance. I can say "when" and proceed with my daily life, by all practical measures, without dementia. Nevertheless, I somehow believe that this little word "when" might help open up a portal of empathy, or understanding.

The year I began saying "when I have dementia" was also the year I began facilitating workshops on dementia and spirituality. At one of these workshops, which was hosted at a local church, I introduced the *if*-to-*when* switch, challenging participants to try this turn of phrase as a gesture toward closing the distance between "us" and "them."

One woman said this new language made her feel less afraid. Another woman angrily approached me at the break. "I refuse to say 'when I have dementia,'" she declared. "I will not claim dementia as inevitable for my life!" When I tried to explain the purpose as lowering psychological barriers and increasing compassion, rather than expressing an actual desire to have the condition (I do not relish my own odds), she cut me off: "You *claim* what you *name*, and I will NOT claim dementia!" Her language struck me as vaguely familiar, as words from some vocabulary I had once known more intimately but could no longer readily recall.

When I recounted the episode to a friend, he responded, "She sounds like Joel Osteen!" Ah yes, that was it. She was preaching a version of the prosperity gospel: if your personal faith is strong enough, you can triumph over all manner of human shortcomings. Any negativity—that is, any concession to human finitude or limitations—supposedly reveals a lack of faith and thus invites negative consequences. The power of positive thinking, in other words, can redeem any predicament.

This particular permutation on the prosperity gospel reflects the Word of Faith movement and its emphasis on the power of the word, spoken by the faithful, to claim personal blessings of health and wealth by speaking them into existence.

Alternately, people can utter "negative confessions," which have the power to produce suffering, illness, and disease. In my estimation, this gospel fails to take into full account one central fact: dying, in all its manifold forms—that we all end up failing, no matter our declared intentions to the contrary.

Even if her theology troubled me, I understood her fear and the impulse to resolve it. If our words can invite or thwart dementia, then we can regain a sense of control—which is more comforting than admitting dementia's unpredictability. Most surveys of the U.S. population indicate that Alzheimer's disease is second only to cancer as the most-feared disease; a 2012 Marist Poll revealed that Alzheimer's had become *the* most-feared disease in America. I am not surprised; I see the signs of apprehension everywhere I turn. I see it in people who want to talk to me about dementia; I see it in the people who do *not* want to talk to me about dementia and quickly change the subject. I see it in the woman who, at another dementia and spirituality workshop I facilitated, stood and declared to the group, after telling a teary story of her father's dying years, that she had herbal pills that prevented Alzheimer's. She would sell them to us at the break. I see fear in the little yellow capsules on the edge of my mom's vanity—turmeric, she explained, to reduce inflammation—to prevent dementia. I see it in my divinity school classmate, who never sat in the same seat from class to class, day to day—a habit, he claimed, would stave off Alzheimer's. I see it in the proliferation of magic ingredients that supposedly prevent dementia: coconut oil, B vitamins, ginseng, folic acid, Chinese club moss. I see it in headlines ("How to Avoid Losing Your Mind to Alzheimer's, Dementia"), book titles (*The Anti-Alzheimer's Prescription*), and infomercials for pills that combat memory loss (Cebria, Procera, Prevagen). I hear it in the apocalyptic language that seems to follow dementia—its threat is equated to that of a "tsunami"; its prevalence is an "epidemic" or "pandemic." I hear it every time Alzheimer's receives the grim award of "disease of the century."

I have not only witnessed the fear of dementia from a distance, but I have felt it myself. I need only reread *Casteel Cousins*, or recall the vivid snapshots of Jack's forgetting. I remember how my stomach twisted when, at my cousin's wedding reception, my grandfather told the table that he grew up at the base of Mount Everest. "Mount Rainier," my uncle corrected. No one laughed; it was serious. I have stared at my own bleak Punnett square—the three of the four boxes that possess the ApoE4 variant, the one box that contains two copies of it. Women comprise two-thirds of the Alzheimer's population, for reasons not entirely explained by our longer life expectancy. According to a 2014 study by researchers at Stanford University School of Medicine, having one copy of ApoE4 elevates the risk for women (but not men) who carry the variant.

Despite the fear—or maybe *because* of it and my desire to confront it—I suppose I have decided to name and claim dementia. Or, perhaps more truthfully, dementia has named and claimed me. I was not seeking such a tangled trajectory. It pursued me, it seems, through the intersection of my family and my work. I simply came close enough, for long enough, for it to touch me and anoint me into a different order. During the years I served as the Gardens' chaplain, the residents in the dementia unit kept drawing and redrawing me, kept searching me and knowing me. Their honesty and affection, their desire to connect in a place beyond words, captivated me. Stripped of their powers to name their reality with the precision of finely spoken words, they claimed me another way—through the astonishing transmissions from their inscrutable hearts.

The more aware I grew of their afflictions, what they too often endure—talked over, treated like children, rushed passed, no longer accounted as individuals but discounted as Alzheimer's "victims"—the more convinced I became that the social response to dementia creates as much suffering as the disease itself. Persons with dementia and their care partners often find themselves forgotten at the exact time when they need the most care. I have seen it happen again and again. Friends and family stop calling; faith communities quietly withdraw; physicians offer little support outside prescriptions; public policy often neglects care needs, opting for sexier spending on research for ever-elusive cures. John Swinton, a theologian of disability and dementia, says the problem is not so much that people forget, it is that *they are forgotten*. The problem isn't simply their deficits—it is our distance. Not only do they, the forgotten, miss the gift of our presence; *we* miss the gift of *theirs*.

But their giftedness is not always easy to see or receive.

I am reminded of another person I regularly encountered on my rounds on the dementia unit. Clara could no longer walk, talk, or swallow. Once a professional singer in her native Italy, she melodically moaned when she heard "Ave Maria" or "Pie Jesu." A peg tube had been inserted into Clara's abdomen for artificial nutrition feedings (something her son, I believe, had insisted upon). She sometimes choked on her own saliva—her face turning red as she coughed violently. Despite the staff's best efforts to protect the feeding tube, she regularly pulled it out and went by ambulance to the hospital to have it reinserted. She contracted infections from this hole in her stomach, from hospitalizations that exposed her to all manner of bugs, and from general frailty.

Clara was always reaching out from her reclining wheelchair as people passed by, extending her good arm and not the contracted one curled up against her breast. She seemed to want nothing less than to touch and be touched. When I stopped long enough, when I came close enough to her, she touched my face. She brushed my cheeks, running her fingers tenderly down my jawline. When I reached back, her cheeks were soft, smooth, and ruddy, like halves of a pomegranate. Her eyes met mine. She often looked searchingly. Eyes wide open, she seemed perpetually surprised. I called her *bella*; I am embarrassed I did not know more of her native tongue. She smiled.

There is a thin line between acknowledging, on the one hand, the good that persists in and through adversity, and on the other hand sentimentalizing someone else's suffering. The former keeps us alive to possibilities for transformation; the latter seems merely to mollify our own discomfort. I wish Clara did not have to endure what she did. Nevertheless, she challenged me and others to pass through her deficits, through the sorrow of her state, to receive her gifts. When her soft fingertips touched my face, the harsh world yielded to utter gentleness. I had seen her touch other staff in this way, and watched their tense brows smooth, as perhaps their churning hearts, like mine, calmed for an instant, too. In her compromised condition, she drew us in and blessed us.

Something like Clara's condition is what, I imagine, Janet Adkins feared. On June 12, 1989, Dr. Kenneth Erickson, a psychiatrist, told Janet that she had Alzheimer's. In a *People* magazine interview shortly after Janet's death, her husband, Ron, recalled, "He talked about how [eventually] I would have to dress her and take her to the bathroom. I don't think that needed to be said. Right then Janet said, 'I want to exit.'" In addition to expressing in writing her wish to end her life rather than allow the disease to progress, Janet Adkins carefully orchestrated her own memorial service, held six days after her death. She selected "The Waking" by Theodore Roethke as one of the readings. The first stanza reads: *I wake to sleep, and take my waking slow / I feel my fate in what I cannot fear. / I learn by going where I have to go.*

Janet was not the picture of "fear"; she seemed focused, not jittery, self-possessed, not nervous. I have read of other women with dementia who pursued Janet's same course; they seem anything but fragile. In May 2014, four years after receiving an Alzheimer's diagnosis, Sandy Bem, a pioneering psychologist in the field of gender studies, ended her life by downing a vial of phenobarbital. Gerda Saunders, a retired college professor, was diagnosed with microvascular dementia in 2010 five days before her sixty-first birthday. In her 2017 memoir, *Memory's Last Breath*, she declares that to spare herself from "zombiehood" and her family years of caretaking, she plans to make a "death trip" to Europe, where physician-assisted suicide is easier to access for persons with dementia. In the United States, as of 2019, Oregon, California, Vermont, the District of Columbia, Washington, Montana, and Hawaii permit physician-assisted dying, but laws require that the patient have a prognosis of six or fewer months to live and be "of sound mind," a set of criteria that excludes many people who have dementia. Some activists are pushing for modifications to these restrictions.

I see in these women's decisions not a visible, frantic fear but an underlying, despairing fear—a fear that points to a highly stigmatized cultural landscape in which heavy judgments are placed upon mental impairment, and the threat of suffering neglect or infantilization is great. I see evidence of a deeply internalized stigma when Saunders imagines her own advanced dementia as "zombiehood" and "an undead existence," deploying a horror-inflected vanishing metaphor. These women did what they thought they must, they went where they had to go. I understand the refusal to cede the world of one's creation and control to a world set upon you— and, likely, against you. As a woman myself, I understand the careful maintenance of self-definitions and self-defenses. I understand their vigilance. I understand their decision, even as I depart.

The fear of becoming like Clara, or becoming whatever nightmare we imagine for ourselves when we have dementia, has a shrinking effect. The threat of impending dementia can reduce our inner posture to a petrified position, reminding me of my crouched body during the tornado drills that were a matter of course in my southeast Missouri public school education. At the repeated sound of short, shrill blasts, we abandoned our normal work to flee our windowed classrooms. We lined the hallways, dropped to our knees, tucked knees into chest, tucked head between knees, placed hands over head. The object was to crunch yourself small—the tighter the ball, the better—and prioritize the protection of the head. Whatever you do, do not lift your head. Nervous giggles escaped from our collective crouch. Even the drills were terrifying.

I am searching for an alternative to such fearful constriction in the face of dementia, an alternative that leads neither to self-delusion nor self-expulsion. I want to find another path through fear, to fling it to the compost heap for its conversion to more fertile stuff. I want to believe the gerontologist Anne

Davis Basting when she says, in relationship to dementia, "We can, though, learn to feel *more* than fear." In the face of dementia, I want to believe our choices do not reduce to naïve denial, grim resignation, or life-ending escape.

Lately, it has occurred to me that one step toward feeling more than fear is to draw up my own advance directive or living will. In my chaplaincy training year in the hospital, I helped dozens of patients fill out living wills, and I signed the sheet as a witness. The patients were usually awaiting surgery and requested assistance in completing their advance directives. As they lay on gurneys in the preoperative holding area, in their anxious moments before an impending procedure, they answered questions regarding their desire for artificial fluids and nutrition, antibiotics, mechanical ventilation, cardiac resuscitation. I always marveled at how unflinchingly clear these patients seemed about what they wanted or did not want in the event of a grave prognosis.

I confessed to a chaplain friend that, despite all the living wills I have endorsed, I have never made my own. She scolded, "Why in the world not?" I suppose I have never possessed the kind of clarity about my life and death that lends itself to checkmarks in boxes. I wish to be spared cruelty, but I have never been so certain on the other stuff—like, when frailty crosses into futility, or what kind of life might be acceptable to me, after all. Filling out a formulaic sheet feels crass—an artless transfer of information about that which resists easy transmission. Is not one's life and death worth a good crack at prose? Of course, this writerly insistence might be another form of evasion, another way around facing fear. Maybe it is as simple as *if I cannot feed myself, I do not want to be fed.*

Nevertheless, I imagine what I might say if I were freed from making selections among a set of customary options. I imagine what I might say if I were freed from dementia's driving dread and nebulous shame, if my living will were more of a vision statement than a checklist. I imagine placing an epigraph from *Leaves of Grass* at my living will's beginning: "I am not to be denied, I compel, I have stores plenty and to spare, / And any thing I have I bestow." I might start the body of it in this way: *As I untangle from this world of memory, I choose—no, I sing myself with dementia. I declare dementia a defiant guest but a guest nonetheless, ordained to purify you and me, to render us thoroughly and finally human. I declare myself fully alive. In my late days with dementia, I do not fade; I do not shrink. I may grow dim, but darkness is no enemy. I burn, but I am not consumed; I am undergoing conversion. I present my body, a living will, a testament to a wide and rambling age beyond the singular self.*

It occurs to me that if I proceed in this way with my living will, then the person who has my power of attorney—my husband at present—may have no idea how to execute it. I imagine him consorting with furrowed-brow doctors, who must translate my charged ramblings into practical power. I would not blame them for cursing my poetic pretensions.

An image will not leave me as I consider this will; it is of the Vietnamese monk who set himself on fire in a Saigon intersection in 1963, an act of total protest to total injustice. A ghastly video clip shows him toppling over, engulfed in flame, still in prayer posture—a charred lotus. Robed monks are prostrated in prayer at his fiery edges. I am drawn to the totality of this demonstration, the transparent passion, the self at once committed and detached.

In *Holy the Firm*, Annie Dillard describes a moth that flew into her candle flame. The moth's thorax and abdomen "began to act as a wick." Flame emerged at the jagged hole where her head once sat. "The moth's head was fire." She burned for two hours.

The writer pivots her attention from the smoldering moth to her students: "How many of you [. . .] which of you want to give your lives and be writers?" All the hands went up, she reports. "And then I tried to tell them what the choice must mean: you can't be anything else." I feel the warm exhalation of a knowing sigh, as Dillard concedes: "They had no idea what I was saying." The moth is an immolating monk, a hollow saint—and so it is for the writer. A conduit for flame, beaming a common message of the body and the soul, the writer comes to her end in obscurity, finds the ash heap.

I want to convey something of my aspiration to this self-giving path, perhaps without some of the overt morbidity. I imagine proceeding with the body of my living will: *I bequeath myself to the world; I have no other behest and no other bequest. When I have dementia, I dedicate my body, head and all, to dark brilliance. I take the moth's arc and cast my body, the whole of it, into fire, for burning, for glow. When my lifted head disintegrates, tumbles to ash, to a heap of*

*scattered gray matter—may flame widen through the jagged hole left by
its departing. May the rest of my body, in concert with exquisite darkness,
become the wick sustaining flame. My purpose fulfilled, may I burn out,
finding fire's end: blown out by wind or a more directed will. After emana-
tion, may I go dark, solitude possessing me entirely. Thus hollowed, you and
I become hallow. When my final flight meets final flame, may this life be as
it always was or wished to be: an offering.*

The body's ending seems to have the same obvious obstacles to interpretation as the beginning. I run the risk of my
executors confusing my desire for life with a desire for a feeding tube. I print a standard advance directive form and rather
vacantly check boxes, tuck it away in a folder next to my pass-
port and social security card. Still, I can't help but search for
guiding stories.

I turn to my journal, looking for guides, and find the only
physical trace that I have read *The Invisible Man*. In deliberate
script, I had copied an exchange between the penniless young
narrator and the old woman who has given him room and board:

"I didn't want to be trouble to anyone," I said.
"Everybody has to be trouble to *somebody* . . ."

The old woman's response strikes me as the mantra of a
compassionate counterculture. I am thinking of Dorothy Day
and the other Catholic Workers who took care of Peter Maurin in the last five years of his life. Maurin—who had declared,
"I can no longer think"—suffered from what his doctors called

the "hardening of the arteries in the brain," a once-common explanation for dementia in the elderly. Day frames Maurin's final years not as the ruination of his legacy but as the completion of the poverty to which he had devoted his life. Day, who called Maurin the St. Francis of his day, asserts: "He has achieved the ultimate in poverty [. . .] He has given everything, even his mind." This final stripping, Day reflects, was not something Peter could do for himself, but was the work of God.

Day speaks to Maurin's particular situation and religious commitments (I doubt she would call dementia, broadly, the "work of God"). I appreciate her larger sentiment—that dementia need not be treated as a curse or soul-robber. More than Maurin's condition, Day laments how others sometimes treated him, especially when he was "talked to with condescension as one talks to a child." Day insists Maurin's presence in the community was not burdensome. "It makes me happy to think how everyone was caring for him," reports Day, "And honored to do so [. . .]" Honored, not burdened.

But exactly how much trouble to be to somebody remains imprecise arithmetic, as imprecise as calculating and conveying my wishes—wishes often obscure, wishes in constant revision. I suppose what I am trying to say is this: I declare my will to live with dementia as an act of protest against a dominant culture that wishes not to be troubled by my presence. I pronounce my body deep in dementia a sign of resistance to a society that sees elders, especially elders with dementia, as burdens.

I wonder: When I have dementia, will I be like Clara, always reaching, always searching for warm skin to bless? Or will I be like Helen, who asks repeatedly where she lives and if she belongs here? Will I be like Rita, who possesses an easy laugh and prays ceaselessly? Will I possess the unflappable self-assurance of Lilly, who remains convinced she will walk again even though she has been wheelchair-bound for years, and who says she could have pursued a romantic relationship with Paul but decided to spurn his advances? (Paul is the family member of another resident, and Paul is gay.) Will I recount a fixed story that seems both fundamental to who I am and also slightly off-kilter, like Di, who tells over and over of her kindly, petite mother who once slapped a woman on the street for making a racist remark? Will I be like James and write poetry? Will I be like Rachel and weep in my hands, mourning the losses too many and too fractured to name? Will I be like Joe and tuck my head in my shirt to retreat from a world that does not recognize me? Will I summon the compassion of Suzanne, who holds the hand of her neighbor when she cries? Will I be like Regina and grow angry and violent, falling down again and again, because I refuse to have anyone touch me while I am walking? Will my perversions become apparent like those of Grace, who sings "God Bless America" in one breath, and in the next, shares the size of dick she prefers (a pornographic eighteen inches)? Will I be like Joanne and sleep the day away?

Will I be like Eileen and grind my teeth? Will I be like Freddy and drink too much and think others are entirely beneath me? Will I have strange and powerful delusions like Virginia, who sometimes believes she is a lioness?

I have attempted accuracy in my description of each person, knowing all people are more than, different from, and irreducible to the signifiers assigned them. Maybe I will be (and *am*) like all of them in some way—in the way we carry a heavy accumulation of little things from those whom we encounter. I wonder what distinctive marks will emerge when I have dementia. And who will note them, who will reckon them significant? Who will wish to walk with me? I am priming my husband for my attempts at wit. They can only land, after all, if I have a receptive audience.

I wonder which of my words will come out all wrong, and which will come out shockingly right and offensively honest. Please do not dismiss, out of hand, the truth in the latter. (When Tim, a resident I had visited at length the day before, saw me coming down the dementia unit hallway, he dropped his head into his hands. "Oh no, not you again!" he blurted. "Are you here to ask me a million questions again?") Which words will get stuck somewhere in neural transit? What if my emotional palate is not large enough to name what I am feeling? And what if your emotional palate is too small to understand my strain and the many meanings of silence? I suppose writing carries the same hazards.

———

When I picture my own possible future with dementia, I find some solace in a parable in which Jesus likens God's realm to a woman who has lost a coin. She lights a lamp and sweeps the entire house until she finds it. Dementia, it seems, requires this kind of committed search. When we become "lost" to ourselves, when our thoughts become obscured and our words vanish, we need others to search for us, to refuse to let us slip into oblivion. Like Clara, we never stop wanting to find and be found by another. Only if you ask, shall it be given; only if you seek, shall you find; only if you knock, shall the door open. Somehow these ideas take on a new meaning in light of dementia; they give me—and perhaps only me—some measure of comfort and hope.

When I have dementia, I do not know what parts of myself will go missing. I do not know what can be retrieved. I will need others to pursue me—to light a lamp and sweep the house, plunging into the tiny cracks and dark corners, rummaging through forgotten spaces, upending the entire house—searching tirelessly until I am found. I will play the searching woman while I can, and soon, perhaps, I will be the coin.

9

Vanitas Still Life

IN THE SPRING OF 2018, I RETURNED TO THE MET TO see *Vanitas Still Life*. Perhaps it is good form to return to where one starts, I reasoned. Nearly four years had passed since I'd left the Gardens in suburban New Jersey and started writing this book in earnest. My setting had changed—I now worked with older adults at a large church on the edge of Harlem— but my passion for the subject had not. The petals of Yoshino cherry blossoms coated my path across Central Park. I had the painting to myself again, save for a European tourist who passed between me and the painting, quickly snapping a picture of the skull. I stared into the head's negative spaces and admired the painting's careful symmetries. The irony does not escape me: a painting meant to point to life's evanescence hangs, centuries after its production, in one of the most prominent museums in the world. It has, in fact, "lasted"; its creator is remembered long after his lifetime. I thought I had registered every object in the picture, having scanned it, left to right, top to bottom, multiple times. But, as I made my final pass, I noticed two books, their titles not visible, one at the feet of each of the philosophers. I smiled. Even our cherished volumes do not escape *vanitas*; they, too, are subject to vanishing.

Art, in its many manifestations, seems to push back against the ephemerality of a single life. The poet and critic Allen Grossman's obituary, which reports that he died from "complications of Alzheimer's disease," also contains his definition of poetry: "a principle of power invoked by all of us against our vanishing." It seems poetry—perhaps, more broadly, the impulse to create—reflects the desire to leave a trace, to outlast our limited lifetimes. In a fundamental way, art is an appeal *against* vanishing. I appreciate my aging poet friend Al's frank admission that, for him, "that's the whole game"—producing something that lasts.

The desire to extend beyond our earthly lives—to resist vanishing—can be good. It can challenge us to transcend the prejudices of a particular historical moment, to "take the long view." It can lead us to a commitment to justice, even when its fruits are not forthcoming. It can motivate us to work on projects for the common good that we may never see completed in our lifetimes. It can lead us, against any immediate satisfaction, to plant trees and write books. *Vanitas Still Life* intimates that the brevity of life, which can end as quickly as a bubble bursts, provides a warning against—rather than an invitation to—vain pursuits.

But too often our clinging to life, especially to fixed notions of what the body and the mind *should* be and do, eventuates in an all-out fight against vanishing, morphing into a perpetual state of war against the inevitability of change. This grasping seems to fuel a toxic self-importance, a childish denial of our limitations, and the vain pursuit of "making our mark" without deep consideration of the nature of those marks. Many people whose work has endured long after their deaths are also those who seemed neither to have kept a death grip on their individual lives nor fixated on securing their personal legacies (e.g., Gandhi, Dr. King, Simone Weil). Even as we try to save our lives, it seems, we lose them; and sometimes, those who lose their lives find them.

This letting go does not have to mean martyrdom, but rather, perhaps it involves cultivating a looser relationship to one's being, to one's current abilities, even to dying. On the morning of the day that Thomas Merton died, he gave a talk at an interfaith monastic conference in Bangkok. After stating he would answer questions about his morning lecture at that evening's panel, he concluded, simply, "So I will disappear." These were the last words he uttered in public. He was found dead in his room later that day, apparently having been electrocuted by a metal fan in his bathroom. The same Merton who wrote of solitude, of "God's afternoon," as one day possessing him so entirely that "no man will ever see me again" was, in a blink of an eye, quite literally gone. Fifty years after his death, his books never move far from my reach.

As the head of Dementia Alliance International, an advocacy group composed of people diagnosed with dementia, Kate Swaffer travels the world to promote education and awareness about dementia. She told me about one occasion when, after she had finished speaking about her dementia to a room full of chaplains, an eager attendee shot up her hand and asked, "What does it feel like for you to know that you are going to die?" Swaffer said she was taken aback, and simply responded: "What does it feel like for *you* to know that *you* are going to die?" The woman did not know how to answer. I can't help but think that how we approach our own mortality is the central question demanding our ongoing attention—in part, so that those of us who are healthy resist burdening those who are sick with the task of grappling with both their death *and* ours.

I spent the final hours of my final day at the Gardens with the fourth-floor spirituality group. A few days before, Mary had helped me plan a party for the group, as we sat together outside the nurses' station. It had been one of Mary's middling days. She had accomplished the task of getting out of bed and helping others get to that morning's group activity, but she was too anxious to join in, opting to stay close to the nursing staff.

"We should have butter cookies," Mary instructed me, "with a little decoration on them, some color, a little sparkle." To drink, it would be best to serve lemonade or "something sparkling." The party should be simple and bright. I followed Mary's instructions and served sparkling lemonade and butter cookies in the shape of butterflies, sprinkled with pink, purple, and white sugar—on napkins with sunflowers on them.

In the photo I have of that day, the room is bathed in afternoon light. Eight of us are seated in a semicircle. Anthea is softly smiling, hands resting in her lap. Wide-grinning Bernice holds a sunflower napkin filled with cookie crumbs. And Mary, sporting a bright red button-down shirt and a long string of gold beads, is raising her foam cup, toasting to the day.

Soon after the party, I filled a small bag with the remaining items from my office, stepped outside into the soft glow of the evening's golden hour, and drove westward home. A few days later, I would move out of state for my husband's new job, but on that final afternoon on the dementia unit, no one was going anywhere. In the photo, I am crouched down beside the women, shoulder to shoulder, one among the others—present and happy.

Now, as the minister of older adults at a church, my work with dementia is more diffuse. There is no "dementia unit." From my new vantage point, I can see more clearly the ease with which people who have dementia disappear from the greater community. Tamara, for instance, was an active participant in the older adult programs at the church, until she could no longer drive due to her cognitive decline. An instant chasm opened between her and the community, as Tamara cannot attend the weekly programs now. A confluence of factors—limited public transit options in her area, daughters who work full-time, a church unequipped to provide regular transportation for frail elders—contribute to the distance. I not only worry about Tamara, but I also worry about the group, which is diminished by her absence.

My church has started a regular social gathering for persons with dementia and their care partners called Memory Café—a concept that originated in the Netherlands in the mid-1990s and spread to the United States in recent years. It's a humble initial effort to create a more inclusive environment. While we will continue to look for ways to stay connected to Tamara and others like her, the fact of the matter remains—that my church, like most institutions, is set up for those who are relatively independent, who can navigate complex physical and social spaces. Most institutions tend to inertia, which means they tacitly adhere to cultural biases, so they possess little will or energy around adapting attitudes and structures to the contours of cognitive impairment. I confess that most of the programs I plan assume a high level of cognitive ability. It is hard to keep in mind the needs of those we don't regularly see. And we don't regularly see the people for whom our communities are not designed. The work of transforming ourselves—our spaces, programs, policies, attitudes, and images—is slow, fragmented, frustrating. But I am convinced that it is worthwhile, because becoming more dementia-friendly will make us, in the end, more human-friendly.

Among my friends, reactions to the word "vanishing" are mixed. Nicki said it evoked a sense of magic and mystery for her; she said it made her feel less afraid of death. Hana thought of deliberate stage acts. Michael spoke of birds, visibly present one moment, and in flight and out of sight the next. Samira mentioned the frost on windows "that is beautiful and changes." Al said "vanishing" evoked the pain of erasure, of the invisibility he has experienced as younger poets he had mentored no longer remain in touch or have even slighted him. My parents also heard erasure in vanishing, saying they have reached the age when they sense a creeping invisibility in public. Of course, these latter associations reflect ageism—and are not magical, mysterious, or inevitable. This is different from the vanishing we all must endure as living creatures—the vanishing my friend Alissa associated with the thin line on the horizon, the eye meeting the end of its powers. Beth, a minister friend, said she thought of Jesus's vanishing, his disappearance from the earth that made way for the Holy Spirit to "come and be dispersed, spread around, decentralized, touching all."

As I write this chapter, it happens to be the week between Ascension Sunday, when the post-resurrection Jesus disappears from the earth, and Pentecost Sunday, when the Holy Spirit arrives in flame. It is a week in the Christian calendar firmly suspended between departure and arrival, the gone and not gone. The writers of the Gospels—the earliest of which was crafted a full generation after Jesus's death—had the difficult narrative task of explaining how someone who had come back from the dead was not still hanging around. In their efforts to provide readers a way to understand the gap, they managed to preserve an exquisite, if peculiar, balance between absence and presence. Jesus is gone—"a cloud takes him out of sight," writes Luke. And Jesus is somehow not gone, as he clothes his disciples with "power from on high," thus becoming dispersed, spread around, decentralized, touching all.

While I cannot make sense of these disappearing acts, I want to embrace the tension between presence and absence as residing at the heart of my faith. The paradox leads me away from a static stance toward myself and others, from dividing everything so harshly. It invites me to behold the world's beautiful and sometimes painful fluidity, and to even welcome its transforming and transformative movements. If slipperiness is integral to my faith—is even part of the divine's *modus operandi*—then the "slipping" of the mind need not be a curse.

The stories surrounding Jesus's death and resurrection seem to point, in the end, to a rather ordinary if underrecognized truth: nothing ever really disappears without a trace. The basic laws of physics tell us that both matter and energy are neither created *nor destroyed*. Ecological processes point to transition,

218 LYNN CASTEEL HARPER

not obliteration. The water cycle, for example, reveals nature's conversionary bent. "How interesting to trace the history of a single raindrop!" writes John Muir in the midst of an afternoon storm in the Yosemite. At the downpour's end, Muir charts the many possible paths of its raindrops: some hasten back to the sky as "winged vapor rising," some are synthesized by plants, some are "locked in crystals of ice," some flow to the rivers and oceans. This organic process proves wondrous to Muir: "From form to form, beauty to beauty, ever changing, never resting, all are speeding on with love's enthusiasm, singing with the stars the eternal song of creation." If the natural course of a single raindrop can inspire such reverence, perhaps, the other transmutations within and around my own body, even those I cannot readily observe, might also be worthy of awe.

Muir is particularly taken by water's formation in Yosemite's clouds, noting that even as they disappear "leaving no visible ruins," "not a crystal or vapor particle of them [. . .] is lost; that they sink and vanish only to rise again and again in higher and higher beauty." It could be that the fractured and scattered bits of ourselves—our thoughts, affections, aspirations, abilities—not a crystal or vapor particle of them is lost, too. The various sinkings and vanishings in our own lives might give rise to ascendant beauty, too. Or, at least, this seems in the realm of possibility. I consider my grandfather's vanishing, which, in part, gave rise to this book. And if he passed to me a genetic propensity to suffer his same fate, then part of him may emerge in me through my "vanishing," which strikes me as a strangely comforting symmetry. Presence made visible in absence, not a crystal or vapor particle lost.

"Vanity" in the Ecclesiastes refrain, "All is vanity," happens to be from the Hebrew word for vapor. All is vapor, then—those particles in passing state between liquid and gas, a secondary suspension between the tide pool and the stars. To vaporize is to dissipate into the tiniest pieces, to make disappear from the naked eye. Vapor, the ephemeral conversion into invisibility, regathers as clouds—Muir's "fleeting sky mountains." Bodies, plants or animals, inhale and exhale vapor—such respiration sustains the circulation of the world's body. How to hold this mystifying economy—not with a sigh of lament or hopeless res-ignation, but with a sense of relief, with a world-ending joy of getting to let go finally. All is passing away; all is passing into; all is passing out of; all is passing. We are subject to the wheel-ing motion of death and life, just like all circuitous things.

This is not to say that the losses we experience should not hurt so much or that the pain is "all in our heads"—or that somehow the transitions and transformations in our lives are undemanding or even readily recognizable phenomena. No one in the depth of grief wants glib comfort of their dying loved one as "just in transition." The conjunctive nature of dementia, however, challenges us to contain multitudes, to live between the gone and not gone, between departures and arrivals—to somehow accept the *ands*. I am convinced that this disposition toward dementia can alleviate some of its stigma and dread—so that on our way to death, we know that vanishing is still life.

Author's Note

I AM AN ENTHUSIASTIC READER AND LEARNER, NOT A scholar. I am deeply indebted to the work of others who produced the many articles, books, podcasts, films, lectures, and websites that have enriched my thinking and feeling about dementia, spirituality, aging, and metaphor. In addition to those sources I have explicitly referenced in my book, I would like to acknowledge a few others whose work has been important to this project: Richard Taylor, Susan McFadden, John McFadden, Rebecca Meade ("The Sense of an Ending"), Jane Thibault, Richard Morgan, Jean Vanier, Nancy Eiesland, Amos Yong, Peter Kevern, Gisela Webb, the bloggers at ChangingAging.org, Marigrace Becker and Momentia, Benjamin Hoste's work on the Old Lead Belt, Malcolm Goldsmith, Sam Fazio, Andrew Walker-Cornetta, Janice Hicks, Kathleen Rusnak, Eula Biss, and Atul Gawande.

Acknowledgments

This book would not exist without my editor, Jonathan Lee, who believed in the project from the beginning. It was an honor to work with him, and with my agent, Chris Clemans.

Chapters of this book were published, in different forms, in *Kenyon Review Online*, *North American Review*, *Catapult*, and *The Orison Anthology*. I am grateful to the editors.

I am thankful for the critical support of a grant from the Barbara Deming Memorial Fund.

I am grateful for a great cloud of friends and mentors, many of whom provided specific help and encouragement related to this project, including Matthew Ellis, Beth Honeycutt, Hana Shepherd, Michael Lamb, Denise Lincoln, Alissa Blechle Quaite, Keeley Bruner, Samira Mehta, Beth Lewis Marchbanks, Jon Milde, Bess Puvathingal, Chris Britt, Jen Sabol, Harvey Stark, Nancy Davis and the Grace Baptist saints, and Diane Lipsett. I want to thank my colleagues and friends at

Seabrook and the Gardens, especially David Bowman and Sr. Donna Gaglioti, MPF. The support of my community at the Riverside Church in the City of New York, especially the Tower League, is invaluable to me.

Thank you to Bill Gaventa for pointing me to resources related to theology and disability, especially to John Swinton's *Dementia: Living in the Memories of God.* I am appreciative to those whose daily work brings about a more just world for persons living with dementia; special thanks to Kate Swaffer and Al Power, M.D., for helping me to redefine dementia and for introducing me to Dementia Alliance International.

I am humbled by and grateful to the people living with dementia who have invited me into their lives. I have changed many of their names in the book to respect their privacy; they reside in my heart.

Thank you to my entire family, especially my parents, Curt and Kathy, for their unwavering care and encouragement. And I offer gratitude to Ryan, my partner and poet, for his boundless love and support.

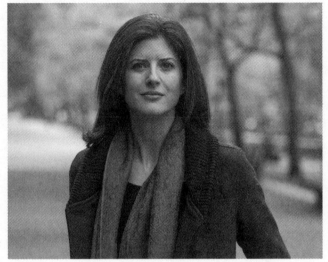

LYNN CASTEEL HARPER is a minister, chaplain, and essayist. Her work has appeared in *Kenyon Review Online*, *North American Review*, and *Catapult* magazine. She is a Barbara Deming Memorial Fund grant recipient and the winner of the 2017 Orison Anthology Award in Nonfiction. She lives in New York City and is currently the minister of older adults at The Riverside Church.